Prevention and Treatment
of
Contraceptive Failure

In Honor of Christopher Tietze

Prevention and Treatment
of
Contraceptive Failure

In Honor of Christopher Tietze

Edited by
Uta Landy

International Women's Health Coalition
New York, New York

and

S. S. Ratnam

Department of Obstetrics and Gynecology
National University of Singapore
Singapore, Republic of Singapore

PLENUM PRESS • NEW YORK AND LONDON

Library of Congress Cataloging in Publication Data

Christopher Tietze International Symposium on the Prevention and Treatment of Contraceptive Failure (1st: 1985: Berlin, Germany)
  Prevention and treatment of contraceptive failure.

  "Proceedings of the First Christopher Tietze International Symposium on the Prevention and Treatment of Contraceptive Failure, sponsored by the International Women's Health Coalition, held September 21–22, 1985, in Berlin (West), Federal Republic of Germany" — T.p. verso.

  Includes bibliographies and index.
  1. Abortion—Congresses. 2. Contraception—Failures—Congresses. 3. Contraception —Failures—Prevention—Congresses. I. Landy, Uta. II. Ratnam, S. S. III. Title. [DNLM: 1. Abortion, Induced—methods—congresses. 2. Abortion, Induced—trends—congresses. 3. Contraception—methods—congresses. 4. Contraception—trends—congresses. W3 C156F 1st 1985p / WP 630 C556 1986p]
  RG734.C47 1985   613.9′4   86-25318

ISBN-13: 978-1-4684-5250-1   e-ISBN-13: 978-1-4684-5248-8
DOI: 10.1007/978-1-4684-5248-8

Proceedings of the First Christopher Tietze International Symposium
on the Prevention and Treatment of Contraceptive Failure, sponsored by the International
Women's Health Coalition, held September 21–22, 1985, in Berlin (West),
Federal Republic of Germany

© 1986 Plenum Press, New York
Softcover reprint of the hardcover 1st edition 1986
A Division of Plenum Publishing Corporation
233 Spring Street, New York, N.Y. 10013

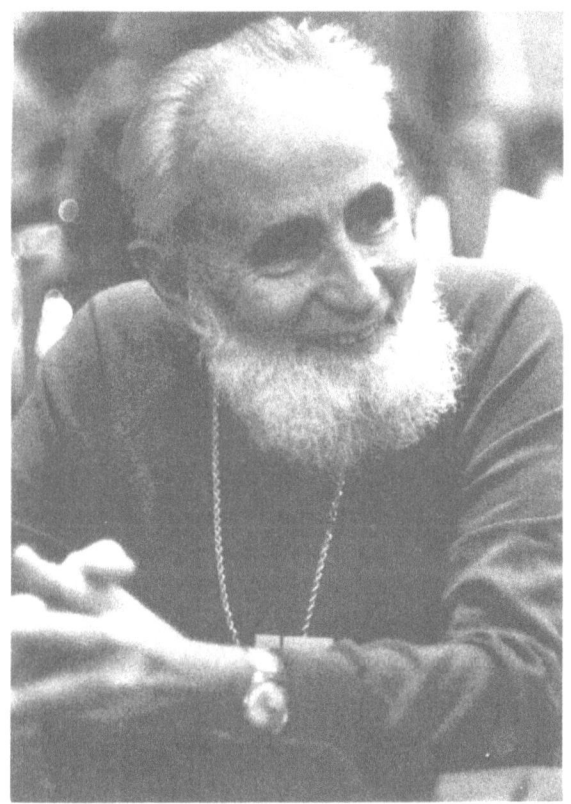

Christopher Tietze, 1908–1984

FOREWORD

The International Women's Health Coalition was pleased to be the convenor and host of the first Christopher Tietze International Symposium, held in Berlin in September 1985. The papers in this volume represent a wide range of international views and experience with the prevention and treatment of contraceptive failure.

We believe the issues discussed at the Tietze Symposium to be of interest and concern to women throughout the world and to those who would serve them. The Coalition intends to give broad distribution to this volume and encourages those interested in these issues to be in touch with the Coalition in New York City (see address below).

We would like to thank The Ford Foundation, Stewart Mott, The David and Lucile Packard Foundation, the Population Crisis Committee, and The Rockefeller Foundation for their support of this Symposium.

In particular we would like to express our appreciation to Sarah Lewit Tietze and Uta Landy for the devotion and dedication which made this Symposium possible and a worthy memorial to Christopher Tietze.

Joan B. Dunlop
President

International Women's Health Coalition
P.O. Box 8500
New York, NY 10150

PREFACE

The death of Dr. Christopher Tietze was a profound scientific, political, and personal loss for the family planning community in the United States and around the world. His scientific brilliance and personal magnetism connected a world community of scholars and activists. Shortly after his death, we began to think of organizing an international symposium to bring together scientists from around the world whom he had influenced and inspired, addressing Dr. Tietze's life-long concerns--the health of women as affected by contraception and legal and illegal abortion around the world. Support for a Tietze memorial symposium came quickly and enthusiastically from individuals, organizations, and foundations. An international advisory committee was established and the International Women's Health Coalition sponsored and hosted the meeting.

The symposium took place on September 21 and 22, 1985, in Berlin (West), immediately following the Congress of the International Federation of Gynecology and Obstetrics (FIGO). It was an inspiring and moving testimony to Christopher Tietze and to all who are dedicated to the health and well-being of women and their families. Those who knew Dr. Tietze personally were gratified to remember him through this international gathering of colleagues, friends, and fellow scientists; others found themselves inspired by the memories and testimonies of those he had taught, advised, or encouraged.

But the meeting did not simply evoke Dr. Tietze's memory; it offered an impressive array of presentations about the health benefits of contraception and safe, legal abortion and menstrual regulation, as well as an international review of social policies and their effect on the health of women and their families. The symposium was so successful that the "Christopher Tietze International Symposia" will be continued as a forum to honor this scientist and present new work in his field.

This publication includes most of the papers presented at the Symposium. They are organized according to subject: prevention of contraceptive failure, effects of illegal abortion on medical practice and public health, medical practice after legalization of abortion, abortion technology, menstrual regulation, delivery of abortion care, maternal mortality in different countries and continents (People's Republic of China, Asia, Africa, South America, Europe, and the United States). These Proceedings begin with a memorial tribute to Dr. Tietze, followed by a worldwide review of information about access to contraception, contraceptive failure, and abortion. The closing presentation takes a global look at the future of women's health.

I want to thank the Advisory Board--Sudesh Bahl Dhall from India, Pouru Bhiwandiwala, George Brown, Allan Rosenfield, Jeannie Rosoff, and Phillip Stubblefield from the United States; Mahmoud Fathalla from Egypt; Evert Ketting from the Netherlands; Fred Sai from Ghana; Benjamin Viel from Chile, and my coeditor, S. S. Ratnam, from Singapore for their invaluable support and guidance. The co-sponsorship of the Population Council, the Alan Guttmacher Institute,

Columbia University's Department of Obstetrics and Gynecology, Assiut University's Faculty of Medicine, the International Federation of Obstetrics and Gynecology (FIGO), the World Health Organization, and the International Planned Parenthood Federation greatly contributed to the success of this meeting, as did the grants of several foundations and individual donors.

My personal friendship and professional admiration for Chris Tietze and his wife, Sarah, who provided encouragement, support, and invaluable help and suggestions during the planning and organization of this memorial symposium, have made my work in preparing the meeting and this publication a source of immense satisfaction. To have known Christopher Tietze and to honor him with this publication is a great privilege.

Uta Landy, Ph.D.
Program Director
Christopher Tietze International Symposium

CONTENTS

MEDICAL PRACTICE AFTER LEGALIZATION OF ABORTION

ABORTION TECHNOLOGY

MENSTRUAL REGULATION: DELIVERY AND TRAINING

DELIVERY OF ABORTION CARE IN HOSPITAL, CLINIC, OR
PRIVATE SETTING: SAFETY, COST, AND ACCESS

MATERNAL MORTALITY

THE FUTURE OF WOMEN'S HEALTH

OPENING REMARKS

    I am greatly honored and highly privileged to have been invited to chair the Christopher Tietze International Symposium on the Prevention and Treatment of Contraceptive Failure. I have had the good fortune to know Chris personally for many years, having sat on the WHO Steering Committee on Sequelae and Complications of Induced Abortion. All of us interested in fertility regulation with particular reference to intrauterine contraceptive devices have heard of Christopher Tietze and of his contributions to life table analysis often related to intrauterine contraception. In the past 10 years he dedicated his professional career solely to research on abortion and published more than eighty articles on this subject. He recognized the limitations of the prevailing methods of contraception, noted that annually some three million unintended pregnancies occurred in the United States and was moved by the grim toll taken of women's physical and emotional health by illegal abortion. He was not afraid to speak or to seek answers to important questions. He was an early and effective advocate of legal abortion in the United States and around the world. His research, prior to the legalization of abortion in the United States and other countries, helped document the subject of clandestine abortion and also the terrible damage it did to women's lives, especially to the lives of those who could not afford or even locate medical practitioners. Once abortion was legalized, Chris monitored the safety with which abortions were being performed, the relationship of the safety to the type of procedure and the period of gestation as he did with intrauterine devices in earlier years. The two major abortion programs in the United States undertaken by the Centers for Disease Control and the Alan Guttmacher Institute were inspired by Chris Tietze and developed with his active assistance.

    His Factbooks on Abortion which he updated almost every year since 1973 are used by all of us interested in this worldwide problem. Not only are they updated reference books, they also contain comprehensive data ranging from laws and policies about abortion to age at which the procedure is performed and the safety and effectiveness of the different methods used today. We should all consider ourselves very fortunate in having had a person of his excellence interested in this field of abortion and its consequences.

    Chris Tietze was born in Vienna where he had begun medical practice in the late 1930s. It was a crucial accident of history that drove him and his family from Vienna to Maryland's shores where he embarked on his career as a biostatistician, demographer, epidemiologist, teacher, advocate, and persuader. His energy, intelligence, curiosity, and passion for justice would never have been satisfied merely with being a private physician for some hundreds of patients when there was so much to be set right in the world and so much that he felt he could do to help set it right.

    As a person he was always kind and friendly. He was always prepared to accept reason and despite his very firm belief in matters related to abortion, he would readily understand and accept the views of others and the situation in other parts of the world. He was an excellent chairman on a number of committees, a friend and adversary; I am happy to have known this exceptionally gifted man.

I have no doubt that this will prove to be the first of a series of such gatherings commemorating this great soul who contributed and published more than any other single individual to our understanding of human reproduction.

S. S. Ratnam, M.D.
Chair
Christopher Tietze International Symposium

President
FIGO (International Federation of Gynecology and Obstetrics)

Professor and Head
Department of Obstetrics and Gynecology
National University of Singapore
Singapore, Republic of Singapore

MEMORIAL TRIBUTE TO DR. CHRISTOPHER TIETZE

Hans Lehfeldt

Clinical Professor
Department of Obstetrics and Gynecology
New York University School of Medicine
New York, New York, U.S.A.

I am honored to join this distinguished gathering of friends, colleagues, and other participants at the "Christopher Tietze International Symposium on the Prevention and Treatment of Contraceptive Failure." I myself am a friend and colleague of many years' standing. I realize that the professional and personal aspects of my memories will inevitably overlap and that neither can stand alone when dealing with a man of Chris's many qualities and gifts. Still, I will try to impart some historical facts and some probably lesser known components of his personality--his warmth and loyalty, his total readiness to give, be it advice, ideas, slides, rare books, or whatever else was needed, and his delightful sense of humor.

Chris and I were introduced to each other by Dr. Robert L. Dickinson in the early 1950s, when Dr. Liebmann and I were evaluating the cervical cap in private practice. Tietze contributed the statistical analysis and Dickinson supplied the illustrations.

A few years later, in 1956, Chris recommended that I conduct a field trial in Barbados of the cervical cap as a contraceptive. My findings were presented at a meeting of the Planned Parenthood Federation, presided over by Alan Guttmacher, and were reported to the United Nations Technical Assistance Program, in both instances thanks to Chris's initiatives.

In the 1960s, Chris and I worked together as members of the Medical Committee, a group of prominent gynecologists which included Drs. Sobrero, Lippes, Guttmacher, Calderone, Garcia, and others.

In May 1960, Chris and I went to Rostock in East Germany as American representatives to the Conference on "Die Internationale Abortsituation, Abortbekaempfung, Antikonzeption" (International Status of Abortion, the Struggle for Abortion, Contraception), organized by Prof. K. H. Mehlan. Crossing the Baltic Sea on a ferry, Chris and I got quite hungry and worried whether upon arriving late in Rostock we would get anything to eat. After all, we were in a country where food was rationed. It was a pleasant surprise when we were greeted at the hotel by a waiter in tuxedo who served us Russian champagne and red caviar.

We were both impressed by the high scientific standards of the meetings, especially by the wealth of new information presented by gynecologists from Czechoslovakia, Hungary, Poland, and Yugoslavia. The data showed that legal abortion is a comparatively harmless operation, less dangerous than tonsillectomy and even less dangerous than childbirth. Tietze's analysis of the data validated these claims and I added the clinical background for a joint-authors' paper which was accepted by the Journal of the American Medical Association (JAMA). To Chris's dismay, some of his analytical statistics were omitted. I tried to comfort him by quoting one of his favorite maxims, "One can't have everything" (Man kann nicht alles haben). This paper and other material was later cited by the U.S. Supreme Court in its 1973 landmark decision legalizing induced abortion in the United States.

Still in the 1960s, Chris and I went to St. Louis for a briefing from Masters and Johnson on their ongoing sex research. While building up his Institute, Masters was then still doing obstetrics and was called away from our meeting to see a patient in labor.

Some time later, I asked Chris to assume an additional workload by becoming the second president of the newly founded Society for the Scientific Study of Sex (SSSS). At the Annual Meeting of the Society, Chris organized a discussion during which legal abortion was freely debated between its advocates and opponents, a daring enterprise in the U.S. in the early 1960s.

The first International Conference on Intra-Uterine Contraceptive Devices was held in New York City in 1962, under the auspices of the Population Council. It was organized by Tietze and Guttmacher and was fundamental in rehabilitating the IUD, a method which had been in disrepute for many years. Gynecologists who had used the IUD for several decades were invited to present their experiences, including Oppenheimer from Israel, Ishihama from Japan, and Lippes, Margulies, and others from the United States.

With the support of the Population Council, Tietze subsequently organized the Cooperative Statistical Program (CSP), a network of statistical and clinical studies to evaluate the safety, effectiveness, and acceptability of IUDs. The Bellevue—New York University Medical Center, where I had founded the Family Planning Clinic, was among the participants. Our participation in this project was a great help in building up and expanding the underfunded family planning clinic. The wealth of material reported by the various cooperative centers was coordinated and evaluated by Tietze. The design of these studies became a standard of perfection for accurate statistical evaluation of contraceptive methods.

One of the many findings was published in 1970 by the American Journal of Obstetrics & Gynecology (AMJOG). The paper "Ovarian Pregnancy and the IUD," authored by myself, Tietze, and Gorstein, was based on data from the multiple participating study centers, and data and slides contributed in reply to our advertisement in AMJOG, inviting reports on ovarian pregnancies with an IUD in situ. We came to the conclusion that the IUD does not protect against ovarian pregnancy.

In 1969, Mary Calderone asked Chris and me to act as co-editors of the second edition of her "Manual of Family Planning and Contraceptive Practice." Chris's own chapters in this book, "Evaluation of IUD Effectiveness" and "The Condom," are masterpieces of scientific writing.

Starting in 1970, Chris became absorbed in the study of abortion, its incidence, its morbidity, its mortality. These studies, known as the "Joint Program for the Study of Abortion" or JPSA, provided the first reliable information on legal abortions in the United States.

Chris was stricken with his first serious illness in 1976, a malignant melanoma which was found during a routine medical checkup and which necessitated a major operation. In case preoperative tests would show metastases, Chris had decided to postpone the operation until he could take care of current commitments. Fortunately, this was not necessary, and he quickly recovered from the operation.

2

In the following year, we both attended a Congress on Perinatal Medicine here in Berlin. Chris had prepared important new mortality statistics on abortion. At the conference, he collapsed and was hospitalized with lobar pneumonia--doubly worrisome because of the ominous possibility of metastases associated with melanoma. When he handed me the slides for his lecture, sick as he was, he was still protesting that he could deliver his lecture himself the following day. Of course, he could not and it took a full week for him to recover sufficiently to return home to New York. I substituted for Chris, presenting his lecture as best I could.

In the face of life-threatening conditions, fully aware of the risks he ran, his characteristic reaction was always the same: he would not stop working nor would he cease to carry out his commitments.

After his retirement, he continued to work as a senior consultant at the Population Council. A few months before his death, he presented a paper at a medical meeting in India and together with his wife travelled for a month through that country--a strenuous enterprise even for a healthy person. We were worried --but Chris was right. He had a most enjoyable trip and he remained well and happy.

However, shortly after his return from India, he was stricken with hemiplegia. On April 4, 1984, he died the way he had wanted it--without a long incapacitating illness and still immersed in his work.

Recognition of his work in the form of celebrations, honors, and awards also gave Chris great pleasure. The tribute which probably pleased him most was the Margaret Sanger award which was given to him and his wife and collaborator. The most unique honor bestowed on him, without doubt, was an official document making him a Kentucky Colonel. He was still with us when the project for a "Christopher Tietze Reproductive Freedom Library" was announced at a special "Toast for Tietze" party. The actual inauguration had to wait until adequate space was found and furnished. The beautiful library was recently installed at Planned Parenthood of New York City.

The two-day International Symposium convened in memory of Christopher Tietze would have given him deep satisfaction, as a tribute to his achievements and as proof that his work of so many years is and will be continued.

AVAILABILITY AND ACCESSIBILITY OF CONTRACEPTION:

A WORLDWIDE PUBLIC HEALTH PROBLEM

Fred T. Sai

Senior Population Advisor
The World Bank
Washington, D.C., U.S.A.

It is a great honor and indeed a privilege to be present at this symposium in memory of one of the stalwarts of international health, Dr. Christopher Tietze. I cannot say that I had the privilege to know Chris Tietze well. Of the three great pioneers in those days, I mention Alan Guttmacher, Bernard Berelson, and Christopher Tietze. I happen to have known Guttmacher and Berelson a little better than I knew Chris. Happily though, by chance I spent a week at the same conference with him in Rehovot, Israel; and on one occasion we had a delightful luncheon chat ranging over many issues. I was profoundly impressed by his dedication to family planning.

It is my view that Chris Tietze was a fighter for the right of everyone to family planning. He chose, like many scientists usually do, to go after the facts, present the facts as he could see them, and let the facts speak for themselves. It is, therefore, only right that in choosing to honor him we should try to follow his lead and let the facts on contraception and abortion speak for themselves.

Since the pill is the method of contraception which created the biggest change in the whole field of family planning, it is perhaps useful for us to remember that the pill has only been in use since the 1960s and that it is constantly being modified. During the last decade, when the pill was subject to a lot of criticism and scare stories in the United States, the U.S. Congress held a hearing. One of the testimonies at that hearing which received very little attention was, in my opinion, a most useful statement. It should be put across the front page of every newspaper to help family planners take courage in the importance of their work as public health work, and to make opponents realize there are women who are mothers, who are physicians, and who know what the pill has done for women in particular and mankind in general. Dr. Elizabeth Connell, formerly associate professor of obstetrics and gynecology at the Columbia University Medical School, in giving evidence before the Nelson Committee on February 24, 1970, stated:

> What has been missing to date, and what I think is needed to maintain an overall proper balance and perspective, is a better look at the vast majority of women who can and are taking oral contraceptives safely and effectively.

> As a physician who began to practice before the advent of the pill, I am constantly aware of the immense difference it has made to the lives of women, to their families, and to society as a whole. The look of horror on the face of a 12-year-old girl when you confirm her fears of pregnancy; the sound of a woman's voice cursing her newborn and unwanted child as she lies

on the delivery table; the absolutely helpless feeling that comes over you as you watch a woman die following criminal abortion; the hideous responsibility of informing a husband and children that their wife and mother has just died in childbirth--all these situations are deeply engraved in our memories, never to be forgotten. Since we have had more effective means of contraception, the recurrence of these nightmares has blessedly become less frequent. The thought that we may once again be forced to face these disasters on an increasing scale because of the panic induced by these hearings strikes horror into the hearts of all of us who have lived through this era once before.

What Dr. Connell is saying about the pill can probably be expressed about practically every family planning method at our disposal today.

It is often recognized, even by people working in family planning, how recent the acceptance by the international community of the right to family planning is. The first official international recognition of the right to family planning came in 1966 when through a unanimous resolution the United Nations General Assembly accepted the principle "that the size of the family should be the free choice of each individual family" (Resolution 221XX).

Other international conferences have since then supported the right to family planning; the two most important have been the Proclamation of Teheran in 1968 and the World Population Plan of Action agreed upon in Bucharest by 136 governments in 1974. The Bucharest conference resolved that "All couples and individuals have the basic right to decide freely and responsibly the number and spacing of their children and to have the information and means to do so. The responsibility of couples and individuals in the exercising of this right takes into account the needs of the living and future children and their responsibility towards the community" (Paragraph 14f, Population Plan of Action).

A right, however, is no right when the people for whom it is meant do not know about it, and do not have access to the enjoyment of it. In many instances it has required legal changes to make it possible for people to have these rights. At the national level there are countries which are establishing specific laws for the provision of family planning information and services. In others, the constitutions themselves have been made to carry reference to family planning as a right for all citizens. Ecuador, Mexico, Portugal, and Yugoslavia are examples. The Chinese constitution includes a reference to family planning but it enunciates its practice as an obligation for citizens rather than as a right.

Despite positive developments, the right to family planning is still the subject of debate and there are governments that withhold information or access for their own ends. It must be affirmed that governments and other authorities on whom society relies have a duty to provide all citizens with the full knowledge about the benefits, purposes and practice of family planning and to make family planning services available to them in as wide a range of methods as possible, including treatment for infertility. Thus individuals and families can make informed choices. And it is during the making of this informed choice that government may have a right through the educational processes to make the individual behavior accord with community or society's needs.

It is my belief that no society has the right to force an individual to behave in support of a government's demographic or economic objectives by withholding family planning information or services.

ACCESS TO FERTILITY REGULATION INFORMATION AND SERVICES

Inherent in the right of everyone to have access to information, education, and services for family planning is the necessity to ensure a wide availability and accessibility of all safe and effective fertility regulation methods. In many societies access is deliberately restricted to some--especially the young and the unmarried. In others some useful methods are withheld. In still others choice is restricted to only one "approved" method--effectively denying access to those not willing or able to use that method.

Apart from such views there are other constraints to the availability of and access to family planning which will be discussed by other speakers at this symposium: the cost of providing fertility regulation services, the type of services within which the provisions are made, the personnel providing the services--these are all factors which could promote or hinder access.

Two major surveys, the World Fertility Survey and the Contraceptive Prevalence Survey, have provided information on contraceptive prevalence for a sufficient number of countries throughout the world to enable us to draw some conclusions.

Most of those using contraception in the world depend on a very small number of methods. Out of nearly 800 million married couples of reproductive age only about 325 million are believed to use effective contraception. One hundred thirty-six million rely on voluntary sterlization, 70 million on IUDs, 55 million on orals, 37 million on condoms, and 30 million on other effective methods (mainly injectables and other barrier methods). Twenty to forty million are believed to use withdrawal, periodic abstinence, or other traditional birth control methods.

Prevalence of contraception varies greatly from region to region, and there are changes over time, too. Needless to say, practice is higher in the more industrialized countries.

The data indicate rapid growth of contraceptive practice during the 1970s in Asia and Latin America. In many cases prevalence increased between successive surveys by over 2 percent and in a few countries by over 3 percent of married women per year. By 1980-1981 at least 33 percent and possibly over 40 percent of women of reproductive age in developing countries including China were estimated to have been practicing contraception. This compares to 66—80 percent of women in most developed countries who are currently using contraceptives. When China is excluded, however, the prevalence rate in the less developed countries drops to only 19—30 percent.

While few African countries have a prevalence rate exceeding 10 percent, recent evidence would suggest Mauritius and Zimbabwe have prevalence rates above 20 percent. Zimbabwe's current rate is estimated to be 22—27 percent. Asia also has wide variations in the level of contraceptive use--from under five percent in parts of South and Western Asia to over two-thirds in some countries of Asia, China, Hong Kong, and Singapore; prevalence is under 5 percent in Afghanistan, Pakistan; 7 percent in Nepal; 13 percent in Bangladesh; and 14 percent in Iraq.

In most Latin American countries at least 33 percent of married women are current users and prevalence rates exceed 60 percent in Costa Rica, Panama, and Puerto Rico and about 50 percent in Jamaica, Trinidad, and Tobago and the lowest, about 20 percent, is seen in Guatemala and Haiti.

Although the differences are not as great in the developed countries, there are substantial differences among the women in contraceptive use. Substantially lower levels of use have been recorded for Japan, Romania, Spain, and Yugoslavia--51—58 percent, while 85 percent of the Flemish women in Belgium are currently using contraceptives. The majority of non-users in the developed countries are considered to be probably either pregnant, immediately post partum, desire to become pregnant, or believe themselves to be infecund. This is not the case for less developed countries where the studies indicate high rates of non-use by women who do not want another child.

From these figures we can draw the conclusion that it is precisely in those countries with poor health services, poor socio-economic development and where needs for contraception are highest that the prevalence rates are really lowest. There is, therefore, a great need for improving family planning services to provide better contraceptive services for a great number of individuals and couples who are in need. It has been estimated worldwide that about 500 million married couples do not have access to efficient contraception despite the knowledge that family planning makes such a tremendous contribution to the reduction of morbidity and mortality of mothers, infants, and young children.

Contraceptives in current use may be classified in many different ways: reversible and irreversible methods of contraception; systemic, and non-systemic. One can use more definitive classifications such as the barrier methods, the pill, the injectables, the IUDs, voluntary surgical sterlization, and natural family planning methods, which should include coitus interruptus. The methods of preventing conception have been adequately described eslewhere and need not concern us at the present time. The only comment I would like to make is that any kind of contraception, however inefficient, is better than no contraception at all. But this is no reason why individuals should not be taught to use the best possible methods available and acceptable in their circumstances.

Some methods of contraception have been subject to a lot of criticism as pointed out in the beginning of this paper.

I would like at this stage, however, to concentrate on voluntary surgical contraception because it has become so popular in the more advanced countries and it is the subject of much misinformation in many less developed countries. In the United States it is the most preferred method, and worldwide, voluntary sterilization protects more women against pregnancy than any other single method of contraception. The incidence is high or rising in many countries and there is no country in which it is declining. In some parts of the world, however--particularly in Africa, but also in some Latin American and Asian countries--the incidence is very low. Puerto Rico and the United States stand out as the countries with the highest sterilization prevalence rates--46 percent and 39 percent respectively. In Europe, the Netherlands stands out with 20 percent and England and Wales with 16 percent. China and India alone, which account for 49 percent of the developing world's population, both have high prevalence rates of 25 and 21 percent respectively. In Africa the only country with any substantial sterilization activity is Tunisia. Some activity is underway in sub-Sahara Africa, but the figures are too small to even count. Practically all sterilization in Africa is of the female, although with increasing effort some small beginnings for vasectomy have been made. In other parts of the world vasectomy accounts for a significant share of sterilization. Asia, China, India, Bangladesh, and Sri Lanka have significant programs of male sterilization. In Great Britain and the United States, the rate of male sterilization is probably among the highest in the world.

Typically, sterilizations in developing countries are accepted more by older people, by people who have completed their family sizes, usually of four, five children or more, while in the developed countries the age range is younger and the family size of the clients is generally two or at most three children.

FACTORS DETERMINING THE USE OF CONTRACEPTION

Age

Contraceptive use patterns differ substantially by age between developed and developing countries. In developing countries, contraceptive use is comparatively low among women aged 30 and younger and rises substantially after that. The greatest period of use is between 25 and 39 years and is seen more in the women in Africa and Asia compared to those of Latin America and the Caribbean.

In the more developed countries, on the other hand, the pattern is relatively even among all married women aged 15 to 24. There is, in fact, a clear tendency for women in most developing countries to use contraception in an effort to stop childbearing altogether rather than for child spacing. Women in developed countries make greater use of contraception to postpone the first birth and to space subsequent births.

Economic Factors

There is considerable variation among countries, even among those with similar gross national products. Guyana, Philippines, and Thailand, for example, have substantially higher levels of contraceptive use than countries with twice the level of GNP per capita. Costa Rica has a high level of contraceptive use--65 percent, although per capita in 1978 of $1,500 was scarcely half the $2,900 in Trinidad, Tobago, and Venezuela where contraceptive use was 52 and 50 percent respectively. The World Fertility Survey data show that some countries are able to achieve higher levels of contraceptive use than others of similar economic status. From the studies by Maudin and Lapham (1985) it has been clearly demonstrated that although social and economic development reinforce contraceptive use and help to increase family planning effectiveness, specific program efforts for family planning are also able to increase contraceptive use. There is therefore no need to put socio-economic improvement as a necessary prerequisite for family planning.

Education

All studies would indicate that education as measured by literacy or number of years of schooling is closely associated with contraceptive use at the national level. Low literacy levels appear to be more of a barrier to contraceptive adoption than low GNP per capita. Widespread contraceptive use is difficult to achieve where literacy levels are low. Except for Haiti, none of the countries where less than 30 percent of adults are literate have contraceptive use levels higher than 10 percent. Contraceptive use increases dramatically as women's years of schooling rise. For instance, Bangladeshi women who have attended school for seven or more years are nearly five times more likely to be contraceptors than women with no education. The finding has been confirmed in many developing countries where regardless of the number of children, the more educated women were more likely to be using contraception than those with less education.

Place of Residence--Rural or Urban

Cross-cultural studies based on World Fertility Survey data have documented the existence of rural versus urban differences of contraceptive practices in developing countries. Generally, the urbanized women use contraception more than women in the country. The reasons are not clear, but it is probably due to a lower awareness of family planning methods, a lack of access to family planning supplies and services and possibly the desire for large families for economic reasons which are more relevant to rural living.

In some countries, such as Malaysia and Guyana, major ethnic groups or distinctive religious groups dominate urban or rural populations, thereby adding the effects of religious and cultural differences. However, in many studies, religious and cultural differences between populations, particularly in the more developed countries, do not seem to provide any basic reasons for the differences in prevalence in contraceptive use. Despite the stand of the Catholic Church, the types of methods used by educated women are similar.

Rural and urban residence has also been found to be related to the type of contraceptive method used by women. For most countries, the urban use of inefficient methods is only two-thirds higher than in rural areas, while the use of efficient methods is on average one to five times higher. Where community based family planning programs have been successful in reaching the countryside, for example, in Indonesia and the Republic of Korea, the use of modern practices is at least as common in the rural areas as in the towns and cities.

Women's Employment Status

The level of fertility is usually negatively related to employment and because contraception is the primary means to control fertility, a relationship exists between contraceptive use and employment status. In the U.S.A. in 1976, women in the labor force were slightly more likely to be using oral contraceptives than other women (Mosher 1981). In some countries, Costa Rica, Jordan, and Korea, the effect of employment on contraception, however, appears to be rather mixed or negligible. This is probably because other confounding variables interact with education, economic, and residence categories and are difficult to separate.

In a recent United Nations study, researchers concluded that it is education, not employment status per se, which accounts for most of the difference in contraceptive use found in the World Fertility Survey.

Law and Regulations

Many countries either have no laws supporting or permitting the provisions of contraception or have specific laws excluding certain methods. In some countries, it is not so much the laws but regulations that are occasionally promulgated by ministries of health which can make for effective access to family planning or block access. Examples are laws and regulations forbidding the provision of family planning services to minors or to unmarried women or those requiring spousal or other consent. Laws and regulations forbidding the performance of voluntary surgical contraception exist in some countries. Most developed countries allow voluntary sterilization for contraceptive purposes. In the U.S.A., Canada, the United Kingdom, and Ireland sterilization for contraceptive reasons is a lawful medical service. Elsewhere in Western Europe, Austria, France, Belgium, Netherlands, and Switzerland, laws have undergone important changes in the last 10–15 years and are now predominantly favorable towards voluntary sterilization. In the majority of Eastern European countries, Bulgaria, Czechoslovakia, and Yugoslavia, either voluntary sterilization is specifically permitted by law or it is not specially prohibited and is by implication allowed. The USSR law is obscure but implicitly negative.

In the developing world over the last 25 years, the nature of legislation on voluntary sterilization has undergone a transformation, although clearly an incomplete one. Increasingly, governments have modified their laws, regulations, and practices to recognize sterilization as an approved method of fertility limitation as distinct from a purely medically necessary procedure for isolated cases, usually women.

But perhaps most important are the actual practices for the provision of contraceptive services. In many developing countries, particularly in Africa, the rules are that family planning services should always be part and parcel of maternal and child health. This, on theoretical grounds, cannot be faulted. However, as the maternal and child health services themselves are reaching only some 20–30 percent of the population in need, such restrictions often mean that contraceptive services cannot be increased prior to a very expensive effort to expand the overall health services. The maternal and child health services themselves need to be reorganized and made more accessible. If that is achieved, integrating contraceptive services would not be too difficult. But there is much to be argued about having contraceptive or family planning services which also help to deliver maternal and child health services.

CONTRACEPTIVE FAILURE

All the contraceptives in use have a failure rate depending on both the efficacy of the method and the user's education and dedication. Surgical sterilization and the injectables have a failure rate of less than one percent; intrauterine devices have a failure rate of 1—5 percent; orals 1—8 percent; condoms 3—15 percent; diaphragms 4—25 percent; spermicides 10—25 percent; and periodic abstinence 10—30 percent.

The issue of how to handle contraceptive failure brings us face to face with that of abortion. Chris Tietze spent much time to provide us with a wealth of factual material to help us make sensible decisions. Despite the complexity of the subject of abortion generally, health workers ought to be exercised about the medical rationale of not assisting when a preventive method has failed through no fault of the user.

ABORTION AND RELATED ISSUES

Abortion has been a major source of controversy from time immemorial. However, in the past few years this controversy has reached dimensions in Western Europe and particularly in the United States which veer on the anarchical. Abortions have been with the world for a long, long time and there is no evidence that abortions will be terminated by legislation. The only evidence we have is that abortions will decrease if effective contraception is used. Abortion can never be completely eradicated. The historical evidence is also strong that rapid fertility decline is unlikely without some recourse to abortion (Corvalan, 1979).

The term abortion simply means termination of a pregnancy after the implantation of the blastocyst in the endometrium, before the fetus has attained "viability," variously defined in law, usually between 24 and 28 weeks. The two major categories of abortions are the induced and the spontaneous. Induced abortions are those initiated voluntarily with the intention to terminate the pregnancy, whether permitted by law or not. All other abortions are called spontaneous.

LAWS AND POLICIES

The legal status of induced abortion ranges from complete prohibition to elective abortion at the request of the pregnant woman. As of mid-1982, 10 percent of the world's four to five billion people lived in countries where abortion was prohibited without exception; 39 percent in countries allowing abortion upon request without specifying the reasons, generally limited to the first trimester of pregnancy; while the remaining 51 percent resided in countries with varying restrictions on abortion.

A large number of countries liberalized abortion laws over the last 15 years. Over the same period four countries in Eastern Europe--Bulgaria, Czechoslovakia, Hungary, and Romania--adopted more restrictive legislation than previously in force. Four other countries--Iran, Israel, New Zealand, and the United States-- liberalized their abortion policies and later made them more restrictive. These experiences have generated a wealth of facts about abortion and health.

SOCIAL JUSTICE

Social justifications for abortion have been the equal access and women's rights arguments, i.e., to give poor women access to services previously available only to the well-to-do, or highly literate, and a postulated right for women to control their own bodies. Another explicit reason in countries like China, Singapore, and Tunisia is to use abortion as one method to curb population growth in the interest of economic and social development.

Opposition to the liberalization of abortion laws has come traditionally from conservative groups, mainly on moral and religious grounds. The Roman Catholic Church has been the most vigorous and articulate opponent. Anti-abortion policies are also favored by fundamentalist Protestants, Moslems, and Orthodox Jews. All of these would maintain that the fetus is a human life right from fertilization despite some of their own theological posits which would argue against such an extreme position.

Concern about low birth weights in subsequent births has been given as a major reason for recent restrictive legislation in Eastern Europe.

Technological advances have made the determination of viability more complex. It is therefore increasingly difficult to use viability as the limit for legal abortion.

INCIDENCE OF ABORTION

The number of pregnancies terminated each year by induced abortion throughout the world is not known, but it has been estimated between 30 and 55 million. The latter figure corresponds to an abortion rate of around 70 per 1,000 women of reproductive age and an abortion ratio of 30 per 100 known pregnancies. Even though no reliable method has yet been developed to estimate the number of illegal abortions, about half of all abortions are considered illegal. More than half of these take place in developing countries. Surveys in some Latin American and Asian countries would suggest as many as one of every three or four women has had an induced abortion sometime in her life. In Africa and the Middle East abortion prevalence seems to be somewhat lower but increasing (Population Reports, 1980). In the major towns of Africa there is evidence that induced abortion is increasing and that among the well educated, abortions are being used increasingly to postpone the first birth rather than for the traditional reason of terminating childbearing.

According to the latest data, the number of legal abortions reported in countries with statistics that are believed to be reasonably complete is almost three million, excluding China, the USSR, and Japan. On a global scale United States women obtain legal abortions at a somewhat higher rate than women in Canada and western European countries, but at a considerably lower rate than do women in Cuba, Japan, the Soviet Union, and most Eastern European nations.

MORTALITY

The earliest nationwide data on mortality following legal abortion originated in Northern Europe where the liberalization of abortion laws began in the 1930s. Data for Sweden indicate a dramatic decline in mortality over three decades—from 250 per 100,000 legal abortions in 1946–48 to 2.4 per 100,000 in 1964–79 (Tietze 1983). In Eastern Europe, Czechoslovakia, and Hungary, levels of mortality during the later 1950s and early 1960s were far lower than those reported for Northern Europe, but even these low rates have declined further in recent years. They reflect virtual limitation of abortion in Eastern Europe to the first trimester. Mortality associated with legal abortion in England and Wales in 1968–69 following the implementation of the Abortion Act was on a level comparable to that achieved in Denmark and Sweden a few years earlier. By the mid 1970s, it had declined substantially. In the U.S.A. following legalization of abortion in New York State in 1970, deaths related to abortion, illegal, legal, and spontaneous, declined sharply by about 51 percent compared to 19 other states with restrictive laws. In the 1970–72 period the decline was substantially less--29 percent. Following the

Supreme Court abortion decision, elective abortion became more easily available to most women and between 1973 and 1975 mortality declined to about three per 100,000 legal terminations, followed by a further drop to about one per 100,000 in 1975–1980 (Tietze, 1983).

Abortion is a major cause of morbidity and mortality in developing countries where the procedure is either illegal or performed under very restrictive laws. Based on a computer model simulating reproductive events, Tietze in 1979 estimated that where most abortions are either self-induced or performed by unskilled providers with poor medical care systems, mortality from illegal abortions could be as high as 1,000 deaths per 100,000 illegal procedures. In most countries, Tietze estimated, mortality, while still high, was probably much lower--perhaps 50 to 100 deaths per 100,000 illegal abortions. In Latin America, where research has been most extensive, even though abortion is illegal everywhere, over 30 percent of maternal deaths in a number of hospitals are due to abortion and related complications (Goldsmith et al., 1970). In Asia and Africa hospitals report that abortion causes between 4 and 51 percent of all maternal deaths.

Apart from backstreet abortions, the risk of death from abortion increases as the number of weeks of pregnancy increases. After 16 weeks, the risk is 25 times higher than the risk before the 9th week, and it is slightly higher than the risk from childbirth. In the United States during 1972–1980 mortality ranged from zero to four per 100,000 legal abortions at eight weeks or less; 14 per 100,000 for abortions at 21 weeks or more. The pattern for abortions without sterilization during 1968–1973 in Great Britain is similar.

Abortion related mortality has appropriately been compared to the risk to life of carrying a pregnancy to term. Deaths related to legal abortion and to childbirth have both declined in many countries over the last two decades, but abortion-related mortality has declined much more swiftly and sharply. In 1970, the mortality rates for the United States were about the same--19 deaths per 100,000 legal abortions and 18 deaths per 100,000 live births. During 1972–1978 mortality associated with childbirth, standardized for age and race, was at least seven times higher than mortality associated with legal abortion combining all gestations (Le Bott et al., 1982).

MORBIDITY

Complications of abortion are more difficult to measure than mortality but are sometimes very common. Worldwide the most frequent complication of legal and illegal abortion is incomplete abortion or retained products of conception. Other major complications are pelvic infection, hemorrhage, shock and trauma to the pelvic organs (cervical lacerations, uterine perforation), and damage to the intestines and bladder. In sub-Sahara Africa and India, tetanus is a major complication and is usually fatal (Akingba and Gbajumo, 1970; Ampofo, 1973).

The legal status of abortion in a country usually influences the specific abortion technique used and thus the subsequent risk to the woman. Where abortion is legal the safest effective technology that is available is usually employed. Where it is illegal, the choice of method is much more limited by the woman's ability to learn of providers, the type of provider accessible, the means at the provider's disposal, and the cost of the procedures. As a result, safety considerations often play little part in determining the method of illegal abortions (Population Reports, 1980). Morbidity, like mortality, varies with the period of gestation. A study of 1,890 women in Santiago, Chile found that 47 percent of abortions performed in the third to fifth month of gestation led to hospitalization compared to 18 percent for those in the first month (Armijo and Monreal, 1965). Similarly, in the United States complications for legal abortions in the second trimester were four to five times higher than in the first (Grimes and Cates, 1979).

LONG TERM CONSEQUENCES OF ABORTIONS

Most of the studies analyzing sequalae of legal abortions do not appear to suggest any long-term impairment of a woman's ability to conceive (Stubblefield et al., 1984; Hogue et al., 1983). Some appear to suggest a higher risk of prematurity, low birth weight, ectopic pregnancies, and spontaneous abortions (Liu et al., 1972; Richardson and Dixon, 1976; Roht et al., 1976). The risks, if any, may be greater for repeated abortions (WHO 1978).

The long term complications of illegal abortion have been more difficult to study. Subfecundity is perhaps the best documented (Trichopoulos et al., 1976). Ectopic pregnancy, premature and still births are all more common in women who have had illegal abortions (Pantelakis et al., 1973).

COST OF ABORTIONS

Illegal abortion is a major public health problem whose costs to women and society are difficult to assess. In some studies from less developed countries 45 percent of all gynecological admissions might be attributed to abortions. Abortion complications comprised 20 percent of admissions to the Maternal and Child Health Institute in Bogota, Colombia (Harrison, 1977), 25 to 57 percent of all gynecological admissions in Nigerian and Ethiopian hospitals (Akingba and Gbajumo, 1970). Extended hospitalization for abortion requires more care and more expensive treatment including blood (a scarce commodity in less developed countries). Direct costs of illegal abortions to women are so high as to consign the poor to use some of the least safe practitioners and methods.

ABORTION AND CONTRACEPTION

Because induced abortion and contraception share the prevention of unwanted or mistimed births as a common objective, a high correlation between abortion experience and contraceptive experience exists in populations where both contraception and abortion are available and in which some couples have attempted to regulate the number and spacing of their children. In such populations, women who have practiced contraception are more likely to have had abortions than those who have not, and women who have had abortions are more likely to be contraceptors than women without a history of abortion (Tietze, 1983).

Among women who do not want to become pregnant, but not all of whom practice contraception, the abortion ratio tends to be high because many unwanted pregnancies are aborted. Women who practice contraception consistently and effectively, however, experience fewer unwanted pregnancies and therefore a lower abortion rate, over a period of time, than those who practice contraception ineffectively or not at all (Gaslonde, 1976).

Although abortion and contraception serve the same purpose, patterns of change over time in the use of these two methods of birth prevention, as reflected by the abortion rate and the rate of known pregnancies based on the sum of legal abortions and of live births six months later, are not at all uniform. A change in the abortion rate may be associated with a change of pregnancy rate in the same direction or with a change in the opposite direction. This apparent paradox is a reflection of the multiplicity of factors determining the rate of known pregnancies.

In some countries pregnancy rates have recently declined over several years in the presence of rising, constant, or declining abortion rates (e.g., Cuba 1972–80; Finland 1976–80; Hungary 1974–80). Such declines in pregnancy rates do not prove, but strongly suggest, wider and more successful contraceptive practices.

Finally, an issue linking abortion and contraception concerns the risk associated with these two methods of fertility regulation. While more than one abortion is required to replace one birth, the risk to life associated with early abortion in a legal setting is much lower than birth-related maternal mortality. Hence, even women who control their fertility exclusively by such abortions are subject, over a given period, to a lower risk of dying from causes related to pregnancy than would be the case if they carried all unwanted pregnancies to term. This is true whether or not contraception is used and probably applies to nonfatal complications as well. It has been conclusively demonstrated that reliance on barrier methods, with early abortion as a back-up, is the safest reversible regimen of fertility regulation for any age (Tietze, 1983).

CONCLUSION

Today family planning is under attack from the industrialized countries as has not been witnessed in the last two decades. Unfortunately the effects of these attacks would be to retard the advances that have been made in the acceptance of contraception, to make effective contraception less readily available and perhaps to force more women towards the less satisfactory option of abortion. In addition to general attacks on family planning, there are those which focus on particular family planning technologies. While some are not perfect, we should not expect a perfect technology. But all family planning methods should be made more accessible to all. Lastly, let me remind you of a good analogy from Malcolm Potts. He compares an individual's needs for fertility regulation to a nation's needs for transportation. No one method is the best for all situations; bicycles and trains have their place, so do bridges and ferry boats.

REFERENCES

Akingba, J. B., Gbajumo, S. A. Procured abortion: Counting the cost. Journal of the Nigerian Medical Association 7(2):17, 1980.

Ampofo, D. A. Epidemiology of Abortion in Selected African Countries. Presented at the IPPF Conference on the Medical and Social Aspects of Abortion in Africa, Accra, Ghana, December 12–18, 1973.

Armijo, R., Monreal, T. The Problem of Induced Abortion in Chile. Milbank Memorial Fund Quarterly 43(4,2):263, 1963.

Corvalan, H. The Abortion Epidemic, In M. Potts, P. Bhiuvandiwala, eds., Birth Control: An international assessment. MTP Press, Lancester, England, 1979.

Gaslonde Sainz S. Abortion research in Latin America. Studies in Family Planning 7:211, 1976.

Goldsmith, A., Gutierrez H., Sanjueza H. Chile, Country Profiles, p 1; 1970.

Grimes, D. A., Cates, W. Complications from legally induced abortion: A review. Obstetrical and Gynecological Survey 34:177, 1979.

Harrison, P. On the septic ward. People 4:12, 1977.

Hogue, C. J. R., Cates, W., Tietze, C. Impact of vacuum aspiration abortion on future childbearing: A review. Family Planning Perspectives 15:119, 1983.

LeBolt, S. A., et al. Mortality from abortion and childbirth: Are the populations comparable? JAMA 248(2):188, 1982.

Liu, D. T. Y., Melville, H. A. H., Martin, T. Subsequent gestational morbidity after various types of abortion. (Letter) Lancet 2:431, 1972.

Mauldin, F., Lapham, R. J. Measuring Family Planning Effort on L.D.C's: 1972 and 1982. In N. Birdsall, The Effects of Family Planning Programs on Fertility in the Developing World. World Bank Staff Working Paper No. 677, The World Bank, Washington, D.C., 1985.

Mosher, W. D. Contraceptive Utilization, United States 1976, Vital and Health Statistics Series 23(7). National Center for Health Statistics, Hyattsville, Maryland, 1981.

Pantelakis, S. N., Papdimitriou, G. C., Doxiadis, S. A. Influence of induced and spontaneous abortions on the outcome of subsequent pregnancies. American Journal of Obstetrics and Gynecology 116:799, 1973.

Population Reports. Complications of Abortion in Developing Countries. Pregnancy Termination, Series F-7, 1980.

Richardson, J. A., Dixon, G. Effects of legal termination on subsequent pregnancy. British Medical Journal 1:1303, 1976.

Roht, L. H., Aoyama, H., Leinen, C., Gallen, P. W. The association of multiple induced abortions with subsequent prematurity and spontaneous abortion. Japanese Journal of Obstetrics and Gynnecology 23:2, 1976.

Stubblefield, P. G., Monson, R. R., Schoenbaum, S. C., et al. Fertility after induced abortion: A prospective follow-up study. Obstetrics Gynecology 62:186, 1978.

Tietze, C. Induced Abortion: A World Review, 5th ed. Population Council, New York, 1983.

Trichopoulos, D., Handanos, N., Danezis, J., et al. Induced abortion and secondary infertility. British Journal of Obstetrics and Gynaecology 83:645, 1976.

United Nations, Fund for Population Activities. Survey of Laws on Fertility Control, New York, 1979.

World Health Organization, Task Force on the Sequelae of Abortion. The association of induced abortion with adverse outcome in the subsequent pregnancy. In J. J. Sciatra, G. I. Zatuchyni, J. J. Speidel, eds., Risks, Benefits and Controversies in Fertility Control. Harper and Row, Hagerstown, Maryland, 1978.

INDUCED ABORTION--A WORLD REVIEW*

Stanley K. Henshaw

Deputy Director of Research
The Alan Guttmacher Institute
New York, New York

INTRODUCTION

One of Christopher Tietze's major activities in his last years was the com-
pilation of international statistics on legal abortion and their publication in a
widely distributed factbook called Induced Abortion: A World Review (Tietze,
1983). When he died, he was working on the Sixth Edition, which was scheduled to
be published in the spring of 1985. Because of the wealth of useful information
about legal abortion that Chris included in the report and the importance of having
recent statistics available in one source, the Alan Guttmacher Institute has undertaken to continue the project. We anticipate that the Sixth Edition will be published in 1986, and we plan to continue to publish updated editions every two years
or so.

The book describes abortion laws and policies in all countries of the world
with populations over one million; the incidence of legal induced abortion in all
countries with available statistics; abortion rates and ratios by the woman's age,
parity, and marital status; statistics on gestation, repeat abortion, and procedures;
statistics and information about complications and mortality; the health and demographic effects of abortion policy; and, new in the Sixth Edition, information on
length of hospitalization and method of payment for abortion services. Most of the
tables include data from all years since legalization, which we have updated with
the most recent years for which data could be obtained.

Below are summarized some of the findings from the new edition.

LAWS AND POLICIES

The availability of legal abortion has continued to expand in recent years.
Since the last Factbook was published, major liberalization of abortion laws has
occurred in Barbados, Portugal, Taiwan, Turkey, and Spain. A liberal abortion law
has been proposed in Greece and is expected to be approved soon. Only one coun-
try--Romania--has seriously reduced access to legal abortion. Also, Ireland has
amended its constitution to make it more difficult for the abortion laws ever to be
liberalized, even though abortion was already illegal in that country. Of course,
legalization of abortion is not the same as increased access. In Taiwan, for exam-

---

* The statistics in this report have been updated with information available to the
author as of April 1986.

ple, abortion services were readily available even before legalization. In India, on the other hand, abortion is legal but most women reportedly lack access to legal abortion services.

Abortion is now legal for broad health reasons in virtually all the countries of Europe, the only exceptions being Belgium, Ireland, Northern Ireland, and Malta. It is also legal in the more developed countries in other parts of the world and in some developing countries, including the most populous ones, China and India. As economic development proceeds and as concern with population growth increases, the most likely prospect is that abortion laws will be liberalized in additional countries.

INCIDENCE OF ABORTION

Abortion rates are stable or declining in all but three of the Western industrialized countries. The abortion rate per 1,000 women aged 15−44 has fallen 20 percent or more from peaks in the 1970s in Denmark, Finland, the Netherlands, and Norway. The rate in the Federal Republic of Germany has also fallen, but the statistics are uncertain because of incomplete reporting of nonhospital abortions. In Canada, England and Wales, France, Italy, Scotland, Sweden, and the United States, rates are stable or are declining slightly. The only countries with increasing rates are Greenland, Iceland, and New Zealand. The generally declining abortion rates suggest that contraceptive practice is improving.

The socialist countries of Eastern and Central Europe, where abortion was legalized earlier, do not conform to the pattern described above. These countries have experienced a number of changes in abortion rates over the years, influenced in large part by fluctuating availability of modern contraceptives and by policy changes to influence population growth. Most recently, rates have been rising slightly in Czechoslovakia, the German Democratic Republic, Hungary, and Yugoslavia, and have been stable in Poland. Rates have been falling in Bulgaria. Rates were fairly stable in Romania before the recent policy changes restricting abortion.

AGE

Abortion rates tend to peak at the age group 20−24. The only exceptions to this pattern are Czechoslovakia and Singapore, where the peak age group is 25−29, and Hungary, where it is 30−34. Teenagers make a substantial contribution to the total abortion rate in the English-speaking countries. Highest is the United States, where 28 percent of the total abortion rate is attributable to teenagers. Also high are Scotland (26 percent), Canada (26 percent), New Zealand (24 percent), and England and Wales (26 percent), as well as Finland (24 percent). Teenagers contribute least, only 7−8 percent in Czechoslovakia and Singapore.

In the most recent three-year period, the contribution of teenagers to the total abortion rate has increased by more than one percentage point in Czechoslovakia, England and Wales, and New Zealand, and has decreased by this amount in Canada, Norway and Sweden.

PARITY

The distribution of abortions by the number of prior births varies widely among the countries. The proportion of abortions obtained by women with no prior births is highest in the English-speaking countries and the Netherlands, where it ranges from 55 to 62 percent, and lowest in Tunisia (7 percent), India (11 percent), Hungary (19 percent) and Italy (24 percent). The remaining countries for which data are available range from 38 to 53 percent. The percentage of women obtaining abortions who have had no children is increasing in about half of the countries and stable in most of the rest. It has been declining only in Canada and Hungary.

In almost all countries, decreasing proportions of abortions are obtained by women who have had four or more children. This may reflect in part the declining numbers of women in the population who have had this many births. It may also reflect the increasing use of sterilization by high-parity women.

MARITAL STATUS

The percentage of abortions obtained by never-married women has been increasing in almost all countries. There are several possible interpretations of this trend, and the explanations may be different for different countries. Among the possible explanations are increasing age at marriage, increasing sexual activity among the unmarried, and changing contraceptive practice either among the married--for example, greater use of sterilization--or among the unmarried.

The countries with the highest proportions of abortions obtained by single women are the United States with 80 percent (this includes previously married women) and Canada with 66 percent. The lowest proportions are found in India (6 percent), Czechoslovakia (13 percent), and Hungary (20 percent).

REPEAT ABORTIONS

The proportion of abortions obtained by women who have had prior legal abortions is increasing in all the countries for which we have data except Hungary. In these countries, it has been only within about the last 10 years that legal abortion rates have reached a level approximating the current rates. Therefore, the pool of women at risk of a repeat procedure is still increasing, and abortion patients are increasingly coming from this pool of women with prior abortion experience.

In the countries for which we have data, the proportion of abortions that are repeat procedures ranges from highs of 49 percent in Hungary and 35 percent in Singapore and the United States to lows of 6 percent in India, 12 percent in New Zealand and 14 percent in France and England and Wales.

GESTATION AND PROCEDURES

The proportion of abortions occurring during the second trimester varies widely among countries, from less than one percent in Czechoslovakia and Italy to about 14 percent in England and Wales and 15 percent in India. These percentages are strongly influenced by policy and system factors as well as by the varying needs of women. Low percentages are frequently caused by legal restrictions on second-trimester abortions and unavailability of services. High percentages may be related to system-caused delay and difficulties encountered by women seeking abortion services.

The distributions of abortions by gestational age have been relatively stable in recent years.

Over 90 percent of abortions are performed by instrumental evacuation, usually suction curettage, in almost all countries. The proportion of abortions performed by uterine surgery--hysterotomy and hysterectomy--has fallen sharply and is now less than one percent in all countries except India.

The proportion of abortions performed along with concurrent sterilization has been in a long-term decline in almost all countries that collect these data. A notable exception is India, where 29 percent of reported abortions were accompanied by sterilization in 1982/83, as compared with 19 percent four years earlier. In the other countries, the proportion of abortions with sterilization ranges from 9 percent in Scotland to under 2 percent in Sweden and the United States.

MORTALITY

Mortality from legal induced abortion has dropped sharply in recent years. Most countries reporting data have achieved a rate of less than one death per 100,000 abortions over the period beginning around 1975. Several countries, including Denmark, Finland, New Zealand, and Norway, have reported no deaths in recent years. The highest legal abortion mortality rate was reported in India, which had five deaths per 100,000 abortions in 1981–1983. It should be noted that while this figure is higher than those of the other countries, it is lower than the rate in the United States as recently as 1971.

SERVICES

The Sixth Edition of the Factbook will present new information on abortion services, including data on the number of nights of hospitalization experienced by abortion patients and sources of payment for services.

The percentage of patients who obtain abortions without staying overnight varies widely, ranging from zero in Hungary to about 94 percent in the United States. Funding of abortion services in most countries is provided through national health plans, which usually treat abortion like any other health care. Thus, in most countries, all abortions are financed through public funds or national health insurance, although some countries require co-payment by some or all patients. However, a few countries, including the United States and until recently, France and the Netherlands, exclude coverage of most abortion services from their national health insurance (Medicaid in the United States). Also, women in some countries such as England and Wales and Poland encounter problems with the government-supported services that lead them to pay for abortion services in private facilities.

CONCLUSIONS

It should be remembered that most of the statistics in the Factbook are derived from the industrialized countries and may not be completely applicable to developing areas. Social and economic conditions are different in each country, and policies and practices relating to abortion must be appropriate to local circumstances.

Nevertheless, it is our belief that almost all countries can learn from the experience of other countries, and that the Factbook contains information to facilitate such learning. Whether one is concerned with the medical aspects of abortion, the delivery of services, the implications of contraceptive practice for abortion, or overall national policy, the experience of other countries can help to put a country's record into perspective and demonstrate the range of possibilities.

REFERENCES

Tietze, C. Induced Abortion: A World Review, 1983. The Population Council, New York, 1983.

Tietze, C., Henshaw, S. K.. Induced Abortion: A Word Review, 1986. The Alan Guttmacher Institute, New York, 1986.

PREVENTION OF CONTRACEPTIVE FAILURE--AN OVERVIEW

Pramilla Senanayake

Medical Director
International Planned Parenthood Federation
London, United Kingdom

ABSTRACT

This paper will focus on the prevention of two aspects of this subject: failure to use contraception and contraceptive failure.

Failure to Contracept

The paper will briefly summarize some of the main cultural, sociological, economic, psychological, and logistic reasons as to why couples, particularly those who wish to plan their families, fail to use contraception. None of the currently available methods of fertility regulation constitute the ideal method, and this paper will assess the existing methods in terms of their acceptability to users around the world.

Contraceptive Failure

Contraceptive failure is usually measured in terms of method failure and user failure. This paper will focus on each in turn, suggesting possible ways of minimizing contraceptive failure and stressing the importance of follow-up care. Another important factor is the need for service providers to help couples select the method which is most appropriate to their needs, given that an unsuitable method is unlikely to be used effectively, or may be regretted later.

Conclusion

More research into new methods of contraception and ways of improving existing methods is needed, both to widen contraceptive choice, and to improve acceptability. Family planning efforts need to be expanded, so that increased availability of contraception is made possible due to a wider reach of programs. Finally, cultural and social constraints need to be overcome through increased support for family planning conceptually, financially, and politically.

PREVENTION OF CONTRACEPTIVE FAILURE

The prime objectives of family planning programs throughout the world are to prevent unwanted pregnancies and to bring about wanted births. The spirit of the Planned Parenthood movement is summed up in the famous slogan "Every Child a Wanted Child." Programs aim to reduce the tragedy of unwanted pregnancies by promoting the widespread, voluntary use of contraceptives, since, in a sense, every unwanted pregnancy represents a contraceptive failure of a sort—either a failure to use contraception or the failure of a contraceptive to work. This paper will analyze some of the main reasons as to why some couples, particularly those wishing to plan their families, do not use contraception. It will also look at reasons for contraceptive failure and will suggest ways in which these setbacks can be minimized and prevention of all types of contraceptive failures can be increased.

Failure to Use Contraception

Using World Fertility Survey data (1984) for 18 countries, it was found that on average, 40 percent of currently married women who wanted no more children were not using a modern method of contraception.

A number of reasons have been put forward to explain why some couples do not use contraception. In some cultures, there is a desire for as large a family as possible, and married couples may feel pressured to begin childbearing early and continue to increase the size of their families as a proof of fertility. In other cultures, husbands feel that the faithfulness of their wives is assured if they are more or less continuously pregnant or breastfeeding. Additional cultural reasons may include religious opposition to family planning or objections to specific methods. Cultural resistance can frequently be lessened by sympathetic programs stressing the health rationale for family planning.

Other reasons for failing to use contraception may be sociological or political, particularly in countries composed of a variety of ethnic groups, where family planning may be feared as a means of altering the sociological composition of the community. Political objections have been raised in developing countries as family planning programs funded by developed country donors are seen as representing "imperialist plots" designed to "keep numbers down" in developing countries so that the American lifestyle, typified by the fact that "one American consumes 40 times what one Indian consumes of the world's non-renewable resources," can be retained. Evidence suggests that this kind of opposition to family planning is on the wane. At the International Conference on Population in Mexico City in August 1984, most developing countries were deeply concerned about the consequences of the U.S. withdrawal of funds to the International Planned Parenthood Federation.

Economic considerations can also prevent couples from using effective contraception. This may be particularly true in countries where large families provide security for old age, additional hands for labor, and other income-generating activities in the meantime. Governments with pro-natalist policies may also provide economic incentives for large families, which may prevent some couples from planning to limit the size of their families.

Couples may also have psychological or logistical reasons for not using contraceptives. Certain methods of contraception may raise psychological worries, for example distrust of the IUD as being a foreign body placed in the uterus and therefore somehow "unhealthy."

Logistical reasons for not using contraception are, in a sense, amenable to improvement, in that problems caused by unreliability of supplies, etc., can be minimized through more efficient program management.

Apart from considerations such as these, the continuing absence of the "ideal contraceptive" is a major reason as to why many couples do not use contraception: even though there is usually a method which is appropriate for couples to use at whatever stage of their reproductive lives, there are disadvantages to each method, and, in some cases, these may constitute sufficient cause not to use contraception. It has been postulated that the ideal contraceptive would be completely safe, effective, free of unwanted side effects, simple to use, cheap, acceptable to all religions and cultures, reversible, not require medical supervision, and not be related to coitus when used. Given this catalogue of qualities, this "ideal contraceptive" is likely to remain elusive for the foreseeable future, if not forever.

It is important, therefore, to evaluate existing methods in terms of their acceptability to users around the world, in order to seek ways of minimizing the failure of couples to use contraception.

Contraceptive Failure

Contraceptive failures are pregnancies occurring in couples who are using contraception and are classified as method failure or user failure. The effectiveness of a given contraceptive method in preventing pregnancy is expressed as the number of pregnancies per 100 users per year (Population Crisis Committee, 1985). Figures currently quoted for all contraceptive methods can be seen in Table 1.

In terms of the prevention of contraception failure, "method failure" rates are only amenable to significant reduction by research and development efforts to improve existing methods and develop new ones. "User failure" rates are more amenable to change. Improved counseling, matching couples with the method most suited to their needs, and providing follow-up care can all improve the extent to which couples use contraceptives consistently and efficiently.

Male and Female Sterilization. Sterilization is the most effective method of contraception, and its acceptability to couples is frequently based on its reliability and the fact that it requires only a single procedure. Acceptability could possibly be enhanced if both male and female procedures could offer reversibility without reducing effectiveness.

Implants and Injectables. Neither implants nor injectables rely on continuing or repeat activities of the user for their effectiveness. Contraceptive failure is rare. The acceptability of both methods relies, to a great extent, on adequate counseling and identification of suitable users. In the case of implants, discontinuation, if desired, requires a repeat visit to a clinic facility and is also time consuming. Injectable users must wait until the effects of the drug wear off.

Table 1: Effectiveness in Preventing Pregnancy
(pregnancies per 100 users per year)

	In Theory (Method Failure)	In Practice (User Failure)
Male Sterilization	0.15	0.2−0.5
Female Sterilization	0.05	0.2−1
Implant (Norplant)	0.3	0.3
Injectables (DMPA)	0.25	1
Intrauterine Device	1−3	1−5
Oral Contraception	0.5	1−8
Progestagen-Only Pill	1	3−10
Condom	1−2	3−15
Diaphragm plus Spermicide	2	4−25
Vaginal Contraceptives	3−5	10−25
Periodic Abstinence	2−5	10−30
Vaginal Contraceptive Sponge	11	15−30

Intrauterine Devices. Again, use-effectiveness of IUDs is high because continuing user motivation and action is not a requirement for contraceptive efficacy of this method. Acceptability may be adversely affected by bleeding problems. Teaching women to feel for the threads of the IUD, to ensure that it is still in place, is important. Selection of IUD users is particularly important in view of the higher risk of pelvic inflammatory disease (PID) for women with multiple partners.

Oral Contraceptives. Oral contraceptives (OCs) are highly effective when they are used properly. Failure rates increase if pills are not taken regularly. The ease of administration, reversibility, and the fact that their use does not interfere with coitus are all major reasons as to why oral contraceptives are so popular. Acceptability drawbacks are mostly the results of reported side-effects, and reports linking OC use with cancer, particularly of the breast and cervix, and an increased risk of cardiovascular disease, particularly to women who smoke. Careful selection of OC users is important, and counseling concerning the need to take pills regularly can minimize contraceptive failure. Counseling is also important in cases where women complain of side-effects such as nausea, breast tenderness, etc. Sympathetic care or possibly switching the woman to another oral contraceptive may minimize the chances of a discontented user discontinuing the use of the pill, thereby risking pregnancy.

Prostagen-Only Pill (Minipill). Available evidence suggests that regular pill-taking is even more important with progestagen-only pills than with combined pills. Acceptability may be increased as, unlike combined oral contraceptives, minipills do not interfere with lactation. However, the increased risk of ectopic pregnancies is a disadvantage. Users need to be aware that the risk of contraceptive failure is higher for progestagen-only pills than for combined OCs.

Condoms. Contraceptive failure for condoms is more likely to be a "user failure" than a "method failure" as condoms are mostly effective if used consistently and properly. Counseling is important in ensuring that couples handle condoms with care and that they know how to prevent leakage and spillage. However, complaints that condom use decreases sensitivity seriously affect the acceptability of this method. This problem is amenable to change as research and development into latex providing greater tactile sensitivity could be undertaken. Most of the recent innovations in condoms have been cosmetic variations in color and shape, but the technology for currently available condoms is not new.

Diaphragms Plus Spermicides. This method of contraception can be effective for couples who use it consistently and conscientiously. Acceptability is adversely affected as it interferes with coitus, and may be seen as being messy. The need for a diaphragm to be fitted by trained medical personnel is an additional drawback. Spermicides may also have an unpleasant taste and smell. As with all barrier methods, contraceptive failure may result from couples "taking risks," and using them inconsistently as a result of the disinclination to use them at all. Research and development into these methods to improve acceptability could prevent many contraceptive failures of this type.

Periodic Abstinence. Periodic abstinence requires the couple to refrain from sexual intercourse during the estimated time of fertility. The extent to which this is perceived as being problematic is directly proportional to the failure rate. The fertile period can be identified by three indicators: the calendar method of recording cycles, measuring basal body temperature, monitoring changes in cervical mucus, or a combination of these. Abstinence may be required for a substantial part of the cycle as the changes in basal body temperature and cervical mucus indicate when ovulation has taken place rather than when it is about to. Consequently, the acceptability of a method requiring no drugs or devices may be offset by the relative lack of reliability and the demands of abstinence. The effectiveness of this method may be improved if an inexpensive, simple test can be developed to predict when ovulation will occur. Contraceptive failures with this method may be minimized if couples are taught precisely what changes in cervical mucus and basal body temperature to look for. Another contraceptive practice can be recommended whereby couples use barrier methods during the fertile period.

Vaginal Contraceptive Sponge. The effectiveness of the sponge, even when used under optimal conditions, ranges from about ten pregnancies per 100 woman-years in parous, highly motivated women to 24 among multiparas in the first year of use. Given that its major attraction is that no medical supervision is required, opportunities for counseling users about correct placement and other aspects of successful use may be limited.

CONCLUSION

More research into new methods of contraception and ways of improving existing methods is needed, both to widen contraceptive choice and to improve acceptability. It is clear that such efforts will not only contribute to reducing "method failure" rates of contraceptives but will also help to minimize "user failure" rates if they improve the acceptability of the methods. This is particularly true of barrier methods of contraception.

Expansion of family planning programs worldwide is also needed to prevent contraceptive failures. This will have the effect of increasing the availability of contraceptive services, which will in turn ensure that programs reach more people. Programs must give counseling and follow-up care a high priority and ensure that the needs of individual couples are matched with the most suitable contraceptive method.

Finally, increased support for family planning is needed at financial, political, and conceptual levels. Financial support is crucial as effective family planning programs, reaching a substantial proportion of given populations, are costly. Political support is necessary, as the views of policy makers, parliamentarians, and indeed the public at large, is crucial for the acceptability of family planning programs. This support for family planning can now be increased with confidence as the need to prevent contraceptive failure is not merely desirable for individual couples. The evidence is now available to show that family planning has a crucial part to play in improving the health of mothers and children worldwide. Today family planning is not only a basic human right. It can be said unequivocally that family planning saves lives.

ACKNOWLEDGMENTS

The author is grateful to Ms. Karen Newman for research assistance provided.

REFERENCES

Population Crisis Committee. Issues in Contraceptive Development Population No. 15, 1985.

World Fertility Survey. World Fertility Survey Major Findings and Implications. International Statistics Institute, Voorburg, Netherlands, 1984.

THE PERMANENT CONTRIBUTIONS OF CHRISTOPHER TIETZE:

METHODS AND MODELS

Irving Sivin

Senior Associate
Center for Biomedical Research
The Population Council
New York, New York, U.S.A.

Christopher Tietze's contributions to reproductive health and human welfare rest on three foundations. These are his systematic, wide-ranging data collection; his lucid, objective analyses of data; and his creative scientific imagination. The latter allowed him to ask significant questions of data and to explore models in quest of answers. Tietze brought his powers to bear on questions of science and of policy with an energy that seemed to increase with the increasing range of his effects.

Tietze was persuaded that public policy should rest on the scientific assessment and interpretation of data. He and his wife, Sarah Lewit, meticulously gathered and analyzed data. The validity of their original observational studies has been repeatedly confirmed (Pierce et al., 1972; WHO Task Force, 1982; Sivin and Stern, 1979). Tietze demanded that data be rigorously scrutinized and interpreted, and that the scope of the data be adequate to address the policy questions which evoked them. He introduced analytic methods, such as the single and multiple decrement life tables, for evaluation of the effectiveness, safety, and acceptability of contraceptives. His imagination provided interpretative models to examine IUD pregnancy rates, ectopic gestation, repeat abortion, and mortality risks of contraception.

In data collection, Tietze pioneered studies of the probability of conception following a single coitus. In the 1950s he examined the effectiveness of barrier methods. In the next decade he organized and orchestrated the demonstration of the safety and effectiveness of IUDs. This required an entire decade of data collection, the cooperation of more than 50 colleagues both from abroad and throughout the United States, and the voluntary participation of 24,000 women. The results brought the IUD into family planning programs.

Tietze relished his data-collecting accomplishments, saying of his vehicle, The Cooperative Statistical Program, that it "has the unique distinction of being the first attempt in the history of contraception to evaluate a new method from the time of its inception ... using a systematic statistical approach" (Tietze, 1970).

The quality of Tietze's data collection and the broader implications of his data-gathering effort to quantify the early medical complications of legal abortion through the Joint Program for the Study of Abortion (JPSA) were characterized by Bernard Berelson as "a model of how a body of valid information can be expeditiously gathered, analyzed and presented as a guide to the formulation of medical and public policy" (Berelson, 1972).

In legalizing induced abortion in the United States, the U.S. Supreme Court cited Tietze's work, data, and interpretations regarding the safety of first trimester abortion. Tietze's later Factbooks on Induced Abortion throughout the world remained faithful to his model of comprehensive data collection focused on policy issues.

Method as well as result mattered to him. Method, in its narrowest sense, implies the forms and procedures--the instruments--which he used in data collection. These instruments with their implied analytic categories were adopted and adapted to fit virtually every subsequent prospective study of the safety and effectiveness of contraceptive methods.

To interpret the data he and others collected, Tietze contributed methods and models in several critical areas. He was the Johannes Kepler as well as the Tycho Brahe of contraceptive effectiveness, formulating the theories of how IUDs functioned as well as diligently observing and recording the performance. In the body of the "Ninth Progress Report of the Cooperative Statistical Program," Tietze formulated the theory that effectiveness of the plastic and steel IUDs he studied was a function of the surface area. He also observed that failure rates associated with IUD use decreased with the increasing age of the user. This observation remained true for the Copper devices as well, but at markedly lower levels (Sivin, 1979). The Copper T 200 has a profile of age-specific accidental pregnancy rates that fits very well the profiles of the Lippes Loop C and D devices. The collared Copper T devices, the TCu 220 C and the TCu 380, however, have failure rates among women under age 25 that are significantly below the pregnancy rates for young users of Loop C or D or of the TCu 200. Among women 35 or over the collared copper devices have had virtually no observed pregnancies. Indeed, the average annual pregnancy rate of the TCu 380, as reported in seven randomized cooperative studies has been about 0.5 per 100.

Tietze examined not only the possible mode of action of IUDs, but also the high proportion of failures that were ectopic. He convinced himself, correctly I think, that the IUD is likely to have effects that are not limited to the uterus alone. Events in the fallopian tubes are affected by IUDs making them protective against ectopic pregnancy.

Let's examine this model statistically. One may take the null hypothesis to be that the IUD works on the uterine level alone and is without effect at the tubal level. The negation of that forms the alternative hypothesis. This may be stated simply: the IUD affects events outside the uterus. To test the null hypothesis Tietze employed three empirical premises. These were:

1.   Normal fecundity of about .20 per cycle is sustained throughout IUD use.

2.   Fecundity is independent from one to another cycle during IUD use unless pregnancy develops.

3.   Of 1,000 fertilizations, three will implant ectopically.

The first premise derives from well–documented work, to which Tietze contributed, on the probability of becoming pregnant during an exposed cycle. The second premise is a conventional statistical device to permit simple calculation of expected values. The empirical content of the third premise derives from hospital-based data from the United States around 1965. It simply mirrors the conditional probability that a pregnancy would implant ectopically. Using these empirical premises, the expected rate of ectopic pregnancy during one year of use can be computed as:

Monthly-Fecundability X Cycles-per-Year X Conditional-Probability-of-an-Ectopic = Expected-Incidence-of-Ectopics;

$$0.2 \ \ X \ \ 13 \ \ X \ \ .003 \ = \ .0078 \ = \ 7.8/1000.$$

Instead of the 7.8 ectopic pregnancies per 1,000 women-years of use, the observations recorded in the Ninth Progress Report showed an ectopic pregnancy rate of only 1.2 per 1,000 women-years of IUD use. This value was significantly lower than the expected value, using the Chi square test. Accordingly, the null hypothesis had to be rejected in favor of the alternative--that IUD has contraceptive effects that are not confined to the uterus.

The observation that IUD-associated ectopic pregnancy rates were 1.2 per 1,000 as opposed to an expected 7.8 per 1,000 (if the IUD had no effect on the tubal level), led Tietze to speculate that in comparison with natural fertility, the IUD provided about 95 percent protection against ectopic pregnancy in each cycle. On an annual basis this works out to be only about 50 percent protection--a relative risk of 0.5. This speculation appears to be correct, insofar as it goes, because Tietze confined his view to cycles which are fertile. The more important case, I believe, involves a comparison with natural fertility. In such a comparison one has to appraise the ectopic pregnancy risks of non-contracepting, cohabiting women. These women, on average, quickly become pregnant but, once pregnant, they are protected against ectopic pregnancy during the course of the (non-ectopic) pregnancy for about nine months. They are also protected while they nurse their infants during postpartum anovulation. For women under age 30, pregnancy rates of the order of 400--550 per 1,000 per year have been frequently observed, rates which are largely dependent on the duration of frequent, unsupplemented breast-feeding. When the conditional probability of an ectopic (.003) as observed in the mid 1960s is multiplied by the pregnancy rate, the expected ectopic rate would range from 1.2 per 1,000 to 1.65 per 1,000. Thus, the IUD would provide only minimal protection (relative risk not less than 0.73 to 1.0) for these women. For older women, age 30 or above, with lower rates of natural fertility, the IUD might not have provided protection against ectopic pregnancy.

Since the publication of the Ninth Progress Report, the total and conditional probabilities of having an ectopic gestation have risen two- or threefold in the United States and Scandinavia, but IUD-associated ectopic pregnancy rates have risen no more than 20--30 percent. Under such circumstances there can be no doubt that the IUD is protective against tubal implantation, and that the devices do not confine their action to the uterine levels. Case control studies indicate that Tietze's contention of a protective effect of the IUD was correct for nonpregnant women (Ory, 1981; Gray, 1985).

One of Tietze's most important models took shape in 1969 (Tietze, 1969), even before the publication of the final report from the Cooperative Statistical Program (CSP). In this model, Tietze estimated the mortality risks associated with no contraception and with various contraceptive methods as well as the risks of induced abortion, both legal and illegal. It was evident to him then that oral contraception, legal abortion, IUDs, and barrier methods were all protective against maternal mortality risks when compared either with no contraception or with illegal abortion. Tietze's analysis showed that barrier methods, backed up by legal abortion, provided the safest path of fertility control. Subsequently, Tietze refined the model, producing age-specific mortality estimates of the risk of contraception (Tietze et al., 1976). These analytic estimates of Tietze are widely incorporated in the labelling of oral contraceptives in the United States today. His research has been literally brought into the homes of millions of users of oral contraceptives.

Christopher Tietze has left us a proud legacy of intellectual zeal, of hard-found facts, and of scientific creativity which we gladly inherit.

REFERENCES

Berelson, B. Foreword to: Joint program for the study of abortion: Early medical complications of legal abortion. Stud. Fam. Plan. 3:97, 1972.

Gray, R. H. A case-control study of ectopic pregnancy in developed and developing countries. In G. I. Zatuchni, A. Goldsmith, J. J. Sciarra, eds., Intrauterine Contraception: Advances and Future Prospects. Harper & Row, Philadelphia, 1985.

Ory, H. W. The woman's health study: Ectopic pregnancy and intrauterine contraceptive devices; new perspectives. Obstetr. and Gynec. 57:137, 1981.

Pierce, A., Hiller, J. M., McGuire, J. Comparison of two large-scale studies of the use-effectiveness of IUDs. Stud. Fam. Plan. 3:205, 1972.

Sivin, I., Stern, J. Long acting, more effective copper T IUDs: A summary of U.S. experience, 1970–1975. Stud. Fam. Plan. 10:263, 1979.

Tietze, C. Mortality with contraceptive and induced abortion. Stud. Fam. Plan. 1(45):6., 1969.

Tietze, C., Bongaarts, J., Schearer, B. Mortality associated with the control of fertility. Fam. Plan. Persp. 8:6, 1976.

Tietze, C., Lewit, S. Evaluation of intrauterine devices: Ninth progress report of the Cooperative Statistical Program. Stud. Fam. Plan 1(55):1, 1970.

WHO Task Force on Intrauterine Devices for Fertility Regulation: Internal IUD Insertion in Porous Women. A randomized multicentre comparative trial of the Lippes loop D, TCu 220 C and the Copper T. Contraception 826:1, 1982.

INTERCEPTION

Jack Lippes

Professor, Obstetrics and Gynecology
School of Medicine
State University of New York at Buffalo
Buffalo, New York, U.S.A.

ABSTRACT

In 1960, Christopher Tietze presented a paper on the "Probability of Pregnancy Resulting from a Single Unprotected Coitus." He determined that the risk varied between one in 25 and one in 50. Couples who engage in intercourse without contraception find that their motivation to prevent pregnancy rises dramatically the next day. They may choose one of two techniques that are effective in preventing pregnancy. Historically the first postcoital contraceptive was oral ingestion of steroids such as diethylstilbesterol (DES) or ethinyl estradiol (EE). This usage was appropriately called "interception." Later, combination steroids were recommended for this purpose, thus reducing both dosage and number of days of drug administration.

A second method of interception available to such patients is the postcoital insertion of an IUD. IUD interception eliminates the nausea that sometimes follows ingestion of such drugs as DES, EE, or a combination of estrogen and a progestin. A postcoital IUD probably prevents pregnancy as late as five or even six days after unprotected coitus, while steroids are useful as interceptives for a maximum of 72 hours.

The choice of which method to use depends on medical history, patient's preference, drug tolerance, the physician's findings on pelvic and physical examination, and finally on good communication between physician and patient. There is a need for public education about interception, especially for adolescents, who produce the largest number of unplanned and unwanted pregnancies.

INTERCEPTION

The woman who has been exposed to unprotected intercourse and wishes to prevent pregnancy has a choice of two methods: (1) postcoital estrogen or estrogen with a progestin, or (2) a postcoital IUD. Postcoital steroids can be used during the first 48 to 72 hours, while the postcoital IUD may well be effective up to six or even seven days after exposure to a possible pregnancy.

Historically, estrogen was first used for postcoital contraception or what is better termed "interception." A large study by Kuchera (1971) demonstrated that diethystilbesterol (DES) was effective in preventing pregnancy after unprotected coitus. DES in 25 mg doses was given twice daily for five days, and it had to be started within 72 hours of unprotected sexual intercourse (Kuchera 1971). In this study, involving 1,000 women, there were no serious drug-induced complications and no pregnancies. However, more than half the patients did have minor side effects, and approximately 50 percent experienced nausea and vomiting. Lehfeldt (1973) suggested that when ethinyl estradiol (EE) was used for interception only 10 percent of patients experienced nausea. Haspels (1973) reported on 2,000 patients successfully using large doses of estrogen to prevent pregnancy. These studies confirm that both estrogen and DES, a stilbene derivative with estrogenic effects, could be used for interception.

Eventually progestins were used for interception (Moggia, 1974). These studies were carried out in Latin America, and progestogens were taken after each episode of sexual intercourse. If, on the average, such a patient took her drug 2 or 3 times per week, it amounted to almost continuous administration and thus progestins may have worked simply by inhibiting ovulation. In the United States, interception is usually an emergency situation. Postcoital estrogen or the IUD is used once but not repeated. Pharmacologically a single dose of steroids would have a different effect, a different mechanism, and perhaps a different result than continuous administration. The pregnancy rate for progestins has been analyzed and was found to be dose dependent (Moggia, 1974). Many failures were reported when a low dose of progestogen was used for interception.

Combined steroids for interception were introduced by Lance and Yuzpe (1977). When EE, 0.1 mg, combined with DL Norgestrel 2.0 mg, were taken in two doses for one day (every 12 hours), the pregnancy rate was calculated to be between 0.0 to 1.9 percent. The reason for this low pregancy rate was probably the easy regimen of taking only two doses of the drug, 12 hours apart. With DES or EE alone, the drug must be taken for a five-day period, a situation requiring greater patient compliance than the two pills per day for one day of combined steroids.

However, the combination of EE plus Norgestrel produces nausea and emesis in 25 percent of patients (Lance, 1977). DES is associated with nausea and emesis in 50 percent of patients (Kuchera, 1971), but only in 10 percent of patients receiving EE (Lehfeldt 1973). As an emergency procedure, the few days of digestive symptoms probably do not inhibit many women from completing even a five-day regimen to prevent pregnancy. However, were this situation to be repeated several times in a year, some patients might not comply with the same consistency seen with the first episode.

Both estrogen and progesterone alter reproductive physiology but the differences are critical in their application to interception. Thus, if progesterone or a progesterone-like compound were used for interception, it could be effective by preventing ovulation (Morris, 1973), whereas estrogen prevents implantation (Morris, VanWegenen, 1973). Progesterone does not accelerate ovum transport when given after fertilization (Morris, 1973). Whether pharmacologic alteration in ovum transport plays any role in interception is questionable. Estrogen has profound physiologic effects when administered after fertilization. For example, it reduces the enzyme, carbonic anhydrase in the female reproductive tract (Board, 1970) (Figure 1). The embryo needs a carbonic anhydrase to excrete its own CO2. Morris (1977) proposed that this explains estrogen's mechanism of action in preventing nidation. The combination pill for interception probably works by a variety physiologic effects, but especially enzyme inhibition.

CATALYZED BY CARBONIC ANHYDRASE

$$H_2CO_3 \rightleftharpoons CO_2 + H_2O$$

Fig. 1

Postcoital IUDs

For interception, a second choice is the insertion of an IUD within six days after unprotected intercourse. Reports confirm the successful use of an IUD insertion as an emergency procedure for interception (Lippes, 1976; Lippes, 1979 Haspels, 1979). In the literature a total of 359 women have been followed and reported the successful use of the postcoital insertion of an IUD for interception. Thus far, no pregnancies have been reported when IUDs have been used for interception.

Time of Cycle

Patients seeking interception tended to aggregate at the middle of the menstrual cycle when chances of becoming pregnant were greatest (Table 1). Older and more educated women generally know the rhythm of human fertility better than less educated and younger women. When unprotected intercourse occurred at midcycle the women realized that the chances of pregnancy were greatest and sought help, which explains the mid-cycle aggregation. Fifty-seven percent of women who sought interception enjoyed the advantage of higher education. There is a correlation between college education and awareness of the services being provided in a community.

Two papers reporting on 299 patients requesting interception found that 88 percent had never given birth (Lippes, 1976; Lippes, 1979). In this group 18 percent had at least one therapeutic abortion. This points to the interesting fact that those who seek interception are young and usually nulliparous. It is not surprising that young women are exposed to pregnancy because of a lack of availability of contraceptives or because of incorrect use of method. Thus the educated are aware that after unprotected coitus something can be done to prevent pregnancy, while the poor and uneducated remain unaware of such medical services.

Only 9 percent of these patients were found to have sperm in their cervical mucus. Sims Huhner tests are usually positive for only 4 hours after intercourse. Patients came in seeking interception between 1 and 7 days after unprotected coitus. Therefore not seeing sperm was not surprising (Table 2). In one study 103 patients were examined for Spinnbarkeit (Lippes 1979). Thirty percent showed cervical mucus that stretched more than 8 cm. This is due to the fact that by the time these patients were seen in the Planned Parenthood center most were postovulatory and their mucus had started to thicken (Table 3).

According to Tietze (1960), the probability of "n" acts of coitus' not resulting in conception is: $p = (25-F)^n/25$, allowing that the average intermenstrual period is 25 days. If we assume one episode of intercourse in a day, then the formula for the probability of not conceiving after a single sexual exposure was developed:

$$p^1 = (25-F)/F \times (25-F-1)/(25-1) \times (25-F-2)/(25-2) =$$

$$(25-F)!/25! \times (25-n)!/(25-F-n)$$

where F is the number of days during which conception can occur. From this formula Tietze determined that the probability of conception after a single episode of intercourse was between one in 50 and one in 25. In a postcoital IUD study that included 299 patients we should have expected at least 6 to 12 pregnancies, if postcoital IUDs did not work. Because these patients aggregated at midcycle, chances of conception were even greater and we should have seen even more than 12 pregnancies. Since no pregnancies occurred, the effectiveness of the postcoital IUD was confirmed.

One-third of the patients who wanted a postcoital IUD had the device removed within 2 months of their insertion because they considered this a single emergency procedure. However, two-thirds of these patients chose to continue the use of the IUDs, demonstrating both a need and a desire to continue contraception.

Table 1: Cycle Day of Unprotected Coitus

Day	Number of Cases	Percent
1–5	5	2
6–9	37	13
10–15	120	44
16–20	64	23
21–28	49	18
	275	100

Table 2: Cycle Day of Exposure in
Sperm-Positive Cases

Days	#	%
1–9	3	17
10–15	11	61
16+	4	22
Totals:	18*	100

* 18 of 81 cases were sperm positive; 63 of
81 cases were sperm negative.

Table 3: Condition of Cervical Mucus
by Spinnbarkeit Length

Cm.	Number	Percent
0.1–4.0	68	66
4.1–8.0	31	30
8.1+	4	4
	103	100

This was an important advantage of the IUD for interception over steroids at the time of this 1979 study. Today we would carefully evaluate nulliparous patients to determine if continued use of an IUD were advisable because of a recently reported relation between IUD use and later sterility (Daling et al., 1985; Cramer et al., 1985). Both these studies reported that monogamous women using IUDs showed no increased risk of developing infertility. Other studies (Ellinor, 1969; Tietze, 1970; Wajntraub, 1970; Zipper, 1971; Tatum, 1975; Erickson, 1976; Kaye, 1977; Sakuraba-yaski, 1977; Vessey, 1978) reported a return to fertility after discontinuing IUD use that is similar to the return to fertility after discontinuing use of a diaphragm.

There was no nausea or dizziness reported with IUD use. IUDs have another advantage in that they can be used for interception up to 6 days after unprotected coitus, while estrogens are not effective after 3 days (Board, 1970, Kuchera, 1971; Lehfldt, 1973; Morris and VanWagenen, 1973; Lippes, 1976; Lippes, 1979). Many of the studies reviewed in this presentation were written prior to 1979. Today, we would first obtain a complete sexual history and would know the number of sexual partners our patients contact. Monogamous patients could be allowed to continue IUD use while those with more than one sexual partner would be advised to use another method. Physicians in 1985 would recommend combination pills, long-term injections, or implants of levonorgestrel steroids (in countries where available), which are contraceptives and also thicken cervical mucus, thus possibly helping to prevent pelvic infections.

There is one advantage to the use of postcoital estrogen to be noted by anyone giving advice on this subject in a Western society: estrogen can be prescribed by telephone whereas an IUD insertion requires an office visit.

SUMMARY OF ADVANTAGES AND DISADVANTAGES OF STEROIDS AND IUDs USED FOR INTERCEPTION

IUDs	STEROIDS
Advantages	Advantages
1. May be effective up to 6 or 7 days after unprotected coitus	1. Ease of administration
2. Minimal side effects, e.g. no nausea or vomiting.	2. Drug may be prescribed by telephone.
3. Leaving IUD in utero allows patient choice of continuing contraception.	3. Less chance of pelvic infections.
4. Low pregnancy rate.	4. Low pregnancy rate.
Disadvantages	Disadvantages
1. Some irregular bleeding.	1. Effective for only a maximum of 3 days after unprotected coitus.
2. Increased risk of pelvic infection.	2. Nausea and vomiting reported with all interceptive formulations.
3. Requires an office or clinic visit for insertion and removal.	3. Not a method for continued contraception.

A review of these studies emphasizes the problem that interception is sought by the older and well educated, while the young adolescent seems to be unaware of the availability of services in their community (Tables 4 and 5). There remains a great need for sex education and adolescent enlightenment about birth control. We can all contribute to fulfilling this task.

Table 4: Education of Patients

	Number	Percent
Education:		
Less than high school	23	10
High School graduate	75	33
Some college	128	57
	226	100

Table 5: Education by Age of Patients

Education by age:

	11-17		18-30		31+	
	No.	%	No.	%	No.	%
Less than high school	14	67	7	4	1	7
High School graduate	4	19	60	31	6	40
Some college	3	14	123	65	8	53
	21	100	190	100	15	100

REFERENCES

Board, J. A. Endometrial carbonic anhydrase after diethylstilbesterol as a postcoital antifertility agent. Am. J. Ob. Gyn. 36:347, 1970.

Cramer, D. W., Schiff, I., Schoenbaum, S.C., et al. Tubal infertility and the intrauterine device. N. Engl. J. Med. 312:941, 1985.

Daling, J. R., Weiss, N. S., Metch, B. J., et al. Primary tubal infertility in relation to the use of an intrauterine device. N. Engl. J. Med. 312:937, 1985.

Ellinas, S. P. Experience with medroxyprogesterone acetate (Depoprovera) as an injectable contraceptive. Int. J. Fertil. 14:275, 1969.

Erickson, R. E., Mitchell, C., Pharriss, B. B., Place, V. A. The intrauterine progesterone contraceptive system. Adv. Planned Parent 11(4):167, 1976.

Haspels, A. A. (University Hospital, Utrecht, Netherlands). (Ectopic pregnancies and IUDs). Personal communication, March 22, 1979. As cited in Population Reports B3.

Kaye, B. M., Reaney, B. V., Kaye, D. L., Eleman, D. A. Long term safety and use effectiveness of intrauterine devices. Fertil. Steril. 28:937, 1977.

Kuchera, L. K. Postcoital contraception with diethylstilbesterol. JAMA 218:562, 1971.

Lance, W. J., Yuzpe, A. A. Ethinylestradiol and d1+norgestrel as a postcoital contraceptive. Fertil. Ster. 28:932, 1977.

Lehfeldt, H. Choice of ethinyl estradiol as a postcoital pill. Am. J. Obstet. Gynecol. 116:892, 1973.

Lippes, J., Maulik, D., Tatum, H. J. The postcoital copper T. Adv. in Planned Parent 11:24, 1976.

Lippes, J., Tatus, H. J., Maulik, D., Zielezny, M. Postcoital copper IUDs. Ad. in Planned Parent 14:87, 1979.

Moggia, A., Beauquis, A., Ferrari, F., Torrado, M. L., Alonso, J. L., Koremblit, E., Mischcler, T. The use of progestogens as postcoital oral contraceptives. J. Reprod. Med. 13:58, 1974.

Morris, J. M. Mechanisms involved in progesterone contraception and estrogen interception. Am. J. Ob. Gyn. 117:169, 1973.

Morris, J. M., VanWaganen, G. Interception: the use of postovulatory estrogens to prevent implantation. Am. J. Ob. Gyn. 115:101, 1973.

Sakurabayashi, M. Experience with polyethylene ring: 1955—1965, part 1. Fertil. Steril. 28:407, 1977.

Tatum, H. J. Intrauterine contraception. Am. J. Obstet. Gynecol. 112:1000, 1972.

Tietze, C. Probability of pregnancy resulting from a single unprotected coitus. Fertil. Steril. 11:485, 1960.

Tietze, C. Fertility after discontinuation of intrauterine and oral contraception. In Proceedings of the 6th World Congress on Fertility and Sterility in Memory of B. Zondik. Fordon & Breach, Science Publications, New York, 1970.

Vessey, M. P., Wright, N. H., McPherson, K., Wiggins, P. Fertility after stopping different methods of contraception. Br. Med. J. 1:265, 1978.

Wajntraub, G. Fertility after removal of the intrauterine ring. Fertil. Steril. 21:55, 1970.

Zipper, J., Medel, M., Pastene, L., Rivera, M., Tatus, H. J. Human fertility control through the use of endouterine metal antagonists of trace elements. In V. Borell, E. Diczfalusy, eds., Control of Human Fertility, p. 199. John Wiley & Sons, New York, 1971.

PREVENTION OF CONTRACEPTIVE FAILURES WITH HORMONAL IMPLANTS

Anibal Faundes

Professor of Obstetrics and Gynecology
Universidade Estadual de Campinas
Campinas, SP, Brazil

Hormonal implants have been in the process of research and development for the last 17 years. Up to the present time the only model which has become a finished product is the NORPLANT(R)* implant system, manufactured by Leiras Pharmaceuticals from Finland under license from the Population Council of New York. A few other models, such as CAPRONOR(R) and a second NORPLANT implant system, are well advanced in the development process.

The NORPLANT system consists of six small Silastic(R) capsules implanted subdermally in the arm by a minor surgical technique. It releases about 70 mcg of levonorgestrel each day during the first year, and around 30 mcg daily from the second year on. This latter dosage corresponds to the amount of the contraceptive steroid administered daily in the minipill. Implants, however, provide constant blood levels of levonorgestrel, as compared with the fluctuating levels observed during use of the minipill, with a peak two hours after the ingestion of a pill and lowest levels at the time of taking the next one (Croxatto et al., 1981; Alvarez et al., 1983; Weiner et al., 1976).

Ovulation is observed in about half of the cycles during use of NORPLANT. Cervical mucus is scanty, thick, and evidences little or no "spinnbarkeit" and ferning. Accordingly, sperm penetration in cervical mucus is very severely impaired. These changes in the reproductive physiology are sufficient to explain its mechanism of contraceptive action; however, it is also known that even during apparent ovulatory cycles, the endocrinology of the cycle is altered in many ways, including progesterone levels significantly below those found in the normal luteal phase (Brache et al., 1985).

The very high effectiveness of the method, which will be discussed in more detail later, is explained by its interference with several aspects of the reproductive process described above, and by the constancy of its action, lack of dependence on the memory or motivation of the user, and freedom from the risk of accidental and inadvertent loss of the device.

The initiation and interruption of use of the method require intervention of medical personnel with appropriate training and moderate manual skill. In many centers, both insertion and removal of the implants are done by nurses.

---

* NORPLANT(R) is the Population Council's registered trademark for contraceptive sub-dermal implants.

The capsules are usually placed under the skin of the inner part of the upper arm, by means of a trocar, with or without the help of a small incision of the skin with a scalpel. Removal is accomplished through a small incision of two to three millimeters, in the site of the insertion. It requires more training and skill than the insertion, but after appropriate training many skillful operators remove the six capsules in five to ten minutes, a time similar to that required for insertion. Both removal and insertion are carried out under local anesthesia. Local reactions are rare, although during the initial experience in a new clinic one or two cases of infection and/or expulsion may be observed before the defective technique is corrected.

For these reasons, it is important that the health personnel who will be responsible for the insertion and removal of the implants are carefully trained.

The low dose of the contraceptive steroid administered with the implants, and the absence of synthetic estrogens in its formulation, make this a method causing much less metabolic disturbance than other hormonal methods, suggesting that the long-term life-threatening risks should also be reduced (Croxatto et al., 1983; Shaaban et al., 1984a; Shaaban et al., 1984b, Shaaban et al., 1984c).

The continuous administration of gestagens, however, together with fluctuating levels of endogenous estrogen, lead to bleeding irregularities ranging from prolonged bleeding to oligomenorrhea in more than two-thirds of the users. The bleeding disturbances are more accentuated during the initial months of use, and slowly improve with time, becoming significantly less frequent after the first year of use, when the daily release has already leveled off at about half the initial dose (Faundes et al., 1978). These changes in the bleeding pattern are by far the most important drawback of the method.

The prolonged periods of bleeding and spotting cause inconvenience to the users, interfere in their sexual life, and provoke the complaint of their partners. Some of the users who are among the one-third who have prolonged bleeding and spotting have difficulty in adjusting to this situation and request removal of the implants. Not surprisingly, bleeding and spotting are the most important reasons for discontinuation of the method.

The amount of blood lost is not increased, because the bleeding is usually light. The hemoglobin levels of the users do not diminish and they may even increase among those who had oligomenorrhea with light periods (Nilsson and Holma, 1981). Bleeding is, thus, not a health hazard, but a rather unpleasant inconvenience that many women (and their husbands) are not ready to tolerate, even if they are informed that the condition will slowly improve with time.

THE HORMONAL IMPLANTS AND PREVENTION OF ABORTIONS

The available hormonal implant system, namely NORPLANT, offers several advantages over currently available contraceptives for the specific purpose of prevention of abortion: they can be used immediately post-abortion, they have a very high effectiveness, and their users do not have the risk of inadvertent and unintended interruption of use.

We will discuss those attributes of NORPLANT implants and the reasons these characteristics are important in the prevention of abortion.

Initiation of Use Immediately after Abortion

Prevention of abortion is based on the avoidance of unwanted pregnancies. As in the case of any other preventive health activity, effectiveness in attaining the desired end, i.e., prevention of abortion, will depend on reaching the population at greatest risk. In this case they are the women most likely to resort to abortion if they become pregnant. Several factors can be identified which are associated with a signicantly greater risk of abortion, but the group with the strongest association and higher relative risk is constituted by women who already have had one or more abortions (Requena, 1968).

Women having an abortion offer particular advantages to preventive actions, because they are easily identifiable, constitute a "captive audience" for information during hospitalization, and are particularly motivated to accept means to prevent further pregnancies. Thus, any program addressed to the prevention of abortion should start by concentrating on this particular group (Hardy and Herud, 1975).

NORPLANT appears to have some advantages over other contraceptive methods for use immediately after abortion, particularly in the case of illegally induced, often infected abortions, so frequent in less developed countries. These patients have an increased risk of thromboembolism, and, consequently, estrogen-containing pills are not indicated, at least during the first week after the abortion (Bonnar et al., 1971). At the same time, intrauterine infection is a contraindication for insertion of an IUD. The progestagen-only low-dose NORPLANT system offers no known contraindication for use immediately after curettage.

Assistance for abortion should be provided in a clinical environment offering the same minimal conditions of cleanliness and asepsis required for implant insertions. Health personnel with the skills and training required for abortion care have the capacity to be trained in insertion and removal of implants. Consequently, NORPLANT is a very good choice for immediate post-abortion contraception, and the consultation for abortion offers a convenient opportunity for NORPLANT insertion.

High Effectiveness

Contraception prevents abortion by avoiding unwanted pregnancy. It is obvious that contraceptive efficiency as an anti-abortion tool is parallel to its effectiveness in preventing pregnancy. The initial multicentered trials comparing the NORPLANT system with the TCu 200 showed the implants to be more effective than the Copper IUD (ICCR, 1978). Subsequently, NORPLANT has been tested in a variety of environments (Shaaban et al., 1983; Satayapan et al., 1983; Marangoni et al., 1983; Lubis et al., 1983), confirming its very high effectiveness, compared to other available methods (Sivin et al., 1983) (Table 1).

No Accidental, Inadvertent Interruption of Use

The subdermal placement of the implants and their location in the arm keep them under easy control of the users. Expulsion of one or more capsules is an

Table 1: Annual and Cumulative Pearl Pregnancy Rates in Population Council Studies of NORPLANT(R) Implants, First Segment of Use

Year	Number of Women Completing Year	Number of Woman-Years		Pearl Rate (Per 100 Woman Year)	
		Annual	Cumulative	Annual	Cumulative
1	778	893.5	893.5	0.3	0.3
2	467	565.9	1,459.4	0.2	0.3
3	383	419.0	1,878.4	0.5	0.3
4	268	308.7	2,187.1	1.3	0.5
5	129	193.5	2,380.6	0.5	0.5

Adapted from: Sivin, I., et al., Studies in Fam. Plan. 14:184, 1983.

exceptional event which will never pass unobserved by the user. This is a great advantage over other methods which require periodic actions by users and providers at more or less fixed times, as is the case for pills and injectables. Interruption of the use of these methods is many times the result of external circumstances, out of control of users and providers. Women may not have the money to purchase the monthly supply of pills or another injection; sickness of a child may hinder a trip to the clinic or supplier on time; the clinic's supplies may be depleted due to logistic problems; or the woman may simply forget to reinitiate use when she should. These are some of the reasons which can cause accidental contraceptive interruptions which are totally unrelated to the woman's intention.

Even with the IUD, partial expulsion or displacement of the device may accidentally and inadvertently occur, resulting in an unwanted pregnancy.

None of these circumstances affect the use of NORPLANT. Users discontinue only at their own will. In practice this means that the effectiveness of the NORPLANT system is the same in the field as in restricted clinical trials. This is not the case for other methods. The importance of this characteristic of NORPLANT for the purpose of preventing abortions is emphasized by the fact that the majority of accidental pregnancies during use of other methods result from forgetfulness or unintended temporary interruption of use.

In conclusion, NORPLANT, and possibly improved hormonal implants yet to be developed, appear to be the reversible contraceptives with the greatest potential for the prevention of induced abortion.

REFERENCES

Alvarez, F., Brache, V., Faundes, A., et al. Levonorgestrel plasma level during continuous administration with different models of subdermal implants. Contraception 27(2):123, 1983.
Bonnar, J., McNicol, G. P., Douglas, A. S.. Blood coagulation and fibrinolysis. In Ronald R. Macdonald, ed., Scientific Basis of Obstetrics and Gynaecology. J & A Churchill, London, p. 207, 1971.
Brache, V., Faundes, A., Johansson, E., et al. Anovulation, inadequate luteal phase and poor sperm penetration in cervical mucus during prolonged use of NORPLANT(R) implants. Contraception 31(3):261, 1985.
Croxatto, H. B., Diaz, S., Miranda, P., Pavez, M. Plasma levels of levonorgestrel in women during long-term use of NORPLANT(R). Contraception 23(2):197, 1981.
Croxatto, H. B., Diaz, S., Robertson, D. N., et al. Clinical chemistry in women treated with levonorgestrel implants. Contraception 27(3):281, 1983.
Faundes, A., Sivin, I., Stern, J. Long-acting contraceptive implants; an analysis of menstrual bleeding patterns. Contraception 18(4):355, 1978.
Hardy, E., Herud, K. Effectiveness of a contraceptive education program for post-abortion patients in Chile. Studies in Family Planning 6(7):188, 1975.
Lubis, F., Prihartono, J., Agoestina, T., et al. One year experience of NORPLANT(R) implants in Indonesia. Studies in Family Planning 14(6-7):181, 1983.
Marangoni, P., Cartagena, S., Alvarado, J., et al. NORPLANT(R) implants and the TCu 200 IUD: A comparative study in Ecuador. Studies in Family Planning 14(6-7):177, 1983.
Nilsson, C. G., Holma, P. Menstrual blood loss with contraceptive subdermal levonorgestrel implants. Fertility and Sterility 35(3):304, 1981.
Requena, M. The problem of induced abortion in Latin America. Demography (2):785, 1968.
Satayapan, S., Kanchanasinith, K., Varakamin, S. Perception and acceptability of NORPLANT(R) implants in Thailand. Studies in Family Planning 14(6-7): 170, 1983.

Shaaban, M. M., Salah, M., Zarzour, A., Abdullah, A. A prospective study of NOR-PLANT(R) implants and the T-Cu 380Ag IUD in Assiut, Egypt. Studies in Family Planning 14(6-7):163, 1983.

Shaaban, M. M., Elwan, S. I., El-Sharkawy, M. M., Farghaly, A. S. Effect of subdermal levonorgestrel contraceptive implants, NORPLANT(R), on liver functions. Contraception 30(5):407, 1984a.

Shaaban, M. M., Elwan, S. I., Abdalla, S. A., Darwish, H. A. Effect of subdermal levonorgestrel contraceptive implants, NORPLANT(R), on serum lipids. Contraception 30(5):413, 1984b.

Shaaban, M. M., Elwan, S. I., El-Kabsh, M. Y., et. al. Effect of levonorgestrel contraceptive implants, NORPLANT(R), on blood coagulation. Contraception 30(5):421, 1984c.

Sivin, I., Diaz, S., Holma, P., et al. A four-year clinical study of NORPLANT(R) implants. Studies in Family Planning 14(6-7):184, 1983.

The International Committee for Contraception Research of The Population Council. Contraception with long-acting subdermal implants: I. An effective and acceptable modality in international clinical trials. Contraception 18(4):315, 1978.

Weiner, E., Victor, A., Johansson, E. D. B. Plasma levels of d-norgestrel after oral administration. Contraception 14(5):563, 1976.

FACTORS CONTRIBUTING TO USE-EFFECTIVENESS

Jacqueline D. Forrest

Director of Research
The Alan Guttmacher Institute
New York, New York
U.S.A.

A major contribution of Dr. Christopher Tietze to the evaluation of contraceptive methods was in the area of application of life-table methodology to study contraceptive effectiveness. Potter (1966) was the first to propose using life tables to calculate the risk of becoming pregnant over a certain time period of use. This was a great improvement over the use of the then commonly used Pearl Index (1932) which produced a measure of effectiveness that did not control for duration of use.

DEFINITIONS OF EFFECTIVENESS

Tietze stressed the difference between the "theoretical effectiveness" of a method, which "refers to the antifertility action of a method or product under ideal conditions" and a method's "use effectiveness," which relates to the experience of a human population with contraception in general or with a particular method or product while exposed to the risk of unintended pregnancy" (Tietze and Lewit, 1968). One would very much like to know the theoretical effectiveness of a contraceptive method, both to evaluate its potential for preventing pregnancy and to identify the extent to which the method itself, rather than a couple's use of it, was responsible for pregnancies among method users. In reality, however, it is only use effectiveness which can be measured. While it is thus impossible to separate pregnancies due to the method and those due to method misuse, use effectiveness measures what actually happens to real users, including effects of problems when using the method appropriately.

MEASUREMENT OF USE EFFECTIVENESS

Three basic pieces of information are needed for each respondent in order to calculate life table measures of contraceptive use effectiveness. They are (1) the method used, (2) the duration of use and/or exposure, and (3) the status at termination of use or at observation. Subcategories of terminal status include user, accidental pregnancy, change of method, discontinuation planning pregnancy, discontinuation because no longer exposed, other discontinuation and loss to follow-up. The use effectiveness of a contraceptive is usually expressed as the percentage of users who did not become accidentally pregnant during the first 12 months of use. In fact, the measure commonly given is not the use effectiveness but the use failure rate, i.e., the percentage of users who did become accidentally pregnant during the first year of use. One can switch readily from one to the other since 100 minus the rate of effectiveness equals the failure rate and vice versa.

The information can be obtained prospectively or retrospectively. In prospective studies, where women are followed over time, chief concerns are unrepresentative loss to follow-up and the influence of being a study participant on the respondent's behavior. For instance, the selection of patients into the study and the extra attention they receive may mean that their motivation and knowledge of how to use the method are greater than would be the case in normal users.

In retrospective studies, where women are asked to report their behavior at certain times in the past, major potential problems are those related to recall and reporting. Women may not accurately remember dates of first and last use. For example, they may forget to report a pregnancy that ended in an early miscarriage or they may prefer not to report a pregnancy that ended in an abortion. For women who are not continually in a regular sexual relationship, it may be difficult to accurately report months of use and nonuse and months when they were having intercourse and when they were not. Most studies therefore deal with currently married women and assume they were continually sexually active except when specifically reported otherwise.

The treatment of multiple method use may affect estimates of use effectiveness. No studies are known which attempt to obtain and use information on patterns of contraceptive use, exposure, and pregnancy by partner for women with multiple partners. Some women do report using more than one method during a specific time period, such as when they use natural family planning to time their use of barrier methods, or using more than one method at a time, such as spermicidal foam and condom simultaneously. In analysis of the U.S. national fertility surveys, the convention has been to classify the woman according to the more effective method used, but the relative rankings of effectiveness have changed from survey to survey.

DIFFERENCES IN USE EFFECTIVENESS

Not surprisingly, studies show differences in rates of use effectiveness. Rates differ by method with some consistently showing higher effectiveness than others. Rates differ from country to country and study to study and rates differ by sociodemographic subgroup within study populations.

Table 1 shows use failure rates, i.e., the percent of women pregnant within the first year of contraceptive use by method used, for the U.S. for 1970–1976. Only currently married women using reversible methods were included. The most effective method was the pill with fewer than 3 percent of women becoming pregnant during the first year of use. The failure rate for the IUD was twice as high and for the condom four times higher. Diaphragm users were five times more likely than pill users to be accidentally pregnant in the first years of use and those using spermicides alone or periodic abstinence were even more likely to become pregnant.

For each group of method users, there was a wide range of failure rates across subgroups. Column 3 of Table 1 shows the range of failure rates calculated for subgroups of age (at beginning of use interval), income, and pregnancy intention. These groups were chosen because these three factors emerged as significant in a proportional hazards life table analysis (see Schirm et al., 1982). Other factors that were tested included age at last live birth, parity, race, religion, education, metropolitan and nonmetropolitan status, region, survey date, and duration of use.

For the pill, the subgroup with the highest failure rate (8.1 percent) was about eight times more likely than the most effective users, of whom 0.8 percent became pregnant. The range for other methods was greater, from a

Table 1. Pregnancies per 100 Women in First Year of Contraceptive Use

	Actual Users	Standardized Estimates	Range
Pill	2.5	2.4	0.8 - 8.1
IUD	4.8	4.6	1.5 - 15.5
Condom	9.6	9.6	0.9 - 35.6
Diaphragm	14.4	18.6	6.4 - 51.6
Spermicides	17.7	17.9	6.1 - 50.2
Periodic Abstinence	18.8	23.7	8.3 - 61.6

Source: Schirm et al., 1982; Grady et al., 1983.

14-percentage-point difference among IUD users to differences of 35—45 percentage points for condom, diaphragm, and spermicide users and a 53-point difference between the best and worst users of periodic abstinence.

These differences are obviously greater than any difference in fecundity by subgroup or difference in theoretical effectiveness would cause. Indeed, Tietze recognized that subgroups with lowest failure rates are the closest observable proxy for theoretical effectiveness and suggested using them as such.

Since use effectiveness varies so widely by subgroup, the type of women using a specific method can influence its observed use effectiveness. This is seen by comparing Column 1 of Table 1, which shows the failure rates of women actually using each method, with Column 2, which shows the estimate of what the failure rates would be if users of each method were the same in terms of age, income, and pregnancy intention. The rates are similar for pill, IUD, condom, and spermicide users, suggesting that users of these methods were similar to the standard population, but diaphragm and periodic abstinence users actually had lower failure rates than estimated for the standard population. This indicates that women choosing to use these methods were more likely than those choosing other methods to be in the subgroups of more effective users.

HOW DIFFERENCES IN USE EFFECTIVENESS COME ABOUT

The use effectiveness of a contraceptive method may vary depending on four types of factors: characteristics of the method itself, the timing of use, correctness of use and other factors affecting method performance. The rate of unintended pregnancy due solely to the characteristics of the method itself would indicate its theoretical effectiveness.

Method

There are reasons why each method of contraception might fail that are independent of how accurately or consistently it is used. For example, the chance of failure of sterilization has been related to the type of procedure used. Various devices used to pinch the tubes closed have been known to sometimes fail in closing the tubes fully or to open after surgery (Soderstrom, 1984).

Clinical studies have shown low estrogen dose oral contraceptives to have slightly higher failure rates than those with higher dosages and the progestin–only mini-pill to have higher failure rates than combination estrogen-progestin formulations (Vessey et al., 1982). Research in the Netherlands suggests that monophasic pills have lower failure rates than biphasic or triphasic formulations (Korteling and Cantel, 1985; Ketting and Leseman, 1986).

The failure rates of sterilization and oral contraceptives are very low and, for orals, the potential influence of other factors is quite great. Although undoubtedly of concern to those couples experiencing unintended pregnancies, the range of method differences in these methods that might affect the chance of failure is so low as to be inconsequential to most users.

Differences in use effectiveness have been found in different types of IUDs (Burnhill, 1985; Liskin and Fox, 1982). Copper and steroid containing devices are generally more effective than inert devices. Effectiveness has also been related to the shape and size of the IUD. Method failure in condoms and diaphragms may be related to holes or tears due to product defects although quality control insures that this is extremely unlikely. Diaphragms and spermicides can form inadequate barriers allowing sperm to pass through the cervix. Johnson et al. (1970) have documented that diaphragms may become dislodged during intercourse so that the cervix is no longer covered. In addition, different brands of spermicides use different strengths of nonoxyl-9 and different formulations of the base carrying it. Clinical tests have shown some differences in effectiveness (Keith et al., 1985) Periodic abstinence can fail because of imprecise prediction of ovulation.

Timing Of Use

The effectiveness of all methods but sterilization is sensitive to the timing of use. The newly available steroidal implants must be replaced after five years, but no user attention at all is required in the interim. Likewise, currently available injectable formulations need no attention between injections, which may be needed as often as monthly. Copper-bearing and steroid-containing IUDs need to be replaced at infrequent intervals ranging from one to four years. Periodic checking insures that the device is still in place. No attention is needed on a constant basis, however.

The other methods of contraception available today require more constant attention. Oral contraceptives must be taken daily for 21 days and resumed again after 7 days, or pills and placebos taken continually. Lower estrogen dose formulations and progestin-only mini-pills have less margin for error in missing one or two days or in varying time of day they are taken (Fraser and Jansen, 1983). The condom, diaphragm, and spermicides are coitus-related and must be used shortly before intercourse. The diaphragm may be inserted some hours before. The spermicide-containing sponge may also be inserted hours before intercourse but long enough to become active. Periodic abstinence methods demand fairly constant attention to various body signs in predicting ovulation and estimating those periods during which intercourse may occur or should be avoided.

Correctness Of Use

It is not enough to use a contraceptive each time one has intercourse. The effectiveness even of sterilization is influenced by such factors as whether the woman was actually pregnant at the time of a tubal ligation or vasectomy. After vasectomy, checks are necessary to insure that sperm are no longer present before the sterilization has actually occurred.

In addition to knowing when to take an oral contraceptive pill, a woman must take them in the correct order. Clinical reports tell of women who became pregnant because they followed the wrong order, going down rather than across rows of pills, for instance. Others tell of women who were confused after hearing that they would have bleeding when they were taking the placebo pills and took those pills instead of the contraceptive when they experienced breakthrough bleeding. Since women may well forget to take a pill at the regular time or for a day or more, they must understand what to do, when and how to take those they missed and whether another contraceptive is needed.

While the IUD works without the woman's intervention, she must check it periodically to insure that expulsion has not taken place. Couples relying on condoms must know when it should be put on and how, as well as the correct way to remove it. They should also know what to do if it does break and have spermicide available in case it is needed.

Diaphragms must be correctly fit and the woman must insure that it is in the right position. Although there is remarkably little information documenting the necessity of using spermicide at all or additional amounts for repeated acts of coitus, its use is virtually universally advised (Wiley, 1985). It must also be left in for a time long enough to ensure that no live sperm remain in the vagina.

To be used correctly, spermicides must be correctly applied, including wetting the spermicidal sponge, shaking some spermicidal foams and filling applicators fully, as well as inserting the sponge, suppository or foam, jelly or cream well into the vagina near the cervix. Couples using suppositories or foam must wait the correct length of time before intercourse for the cervix to become covered with spermicide. If intercourse is repeated, all but the sponge require repeated application of spermicide.

The effectiveness of periodic abstinence is related both to the timing of intercourse within the "safe" period and to the accuracy of the observations of body signs and their interpretation.

Other

Some other factors may intervene to affect the effectiveness of a contraceptive. Vomiting or diarrhea in a pill user may negate the effects of having taken the pill. Some drugs, such as the antibiotics ampicillin and tetracycline, may interfere with pill effectiveness (Fraser and Jansen, 1983; Orme et al., 1984). Possible drug interactions interfering with effectiveness have also been suggested to occur among those using the IUD and spermicides (Simon et al., 1984) Changes in timing of ovulation and the length of the menstrual cycle can affect the accuracy of calculations needed by users of periodic abstinence to estimate "safe" periods.

WHY DIFFERENCES IN USE EFFECTIVENESS OCCUR

While the factors outlined above explain how differences in use effectiveness occur, they do not explain why they happen. Such factors can be grouped into three broad categories--provider, relationship, and personal factors. The personal factors include sociodemographic, psychological, economic, and cultural factors. These factors operate primarily through the timing of use and correctness of use although in some cases they do influence the method and other factors.

Provider Factors

The accessibility of a provider of contraceptive services influences the motivation needed to obtain those services. It also affects the degree to which users will be able to surmount barriers to obtaining a method they want or be put off from using a provider or method because it was inaccessible. Factors related to accessiblity include the provider location, hours, waiting time for appointment or service at the provider and cost. They also include whether the provider offers a specific method. In the United States, for instance, the pill, IUD and diaphragm can only be obtained by making a visit to a physician or a clinic. Clinics provide all methods of contraception, but while all obstetrician-gynecologists provide contraceptives, only 84 percent of general and family practitioners do so (Orr and Forrest, 1985). Private physicians rarely provide condoms or spermicides and, among those providing contraceptive services to adolescents, 90 percent prescribe the pill but only 61 percent fit diaphragms (Orr, 1984).

Approachability is another provider factor influencing method use effectiveness. Such factors as the image of the provider and the provisions for confidentiality, as well as the accessibility factors mentioned above, influence whether the couple has supplies available when it needs them and whether both parties know and understand how to use the method.

The quality of the provider can also influence use effectiveness in fairly direct ways. The skill with which a sterilization is performed or an IUD is inserted is related to the methods' effectiveness. Likewise the information given by the provider about how and when to use the method influences the accuracy of use. For years, for example, many unintended pregnancies among those practicing periodic abstinence were related not to a lack of effort or vigilence but to the fact that marriage manuals describing the method taught that the safe period was midway through the cycle, when ovulation occurs as we now know. The types of followup undertaken by the provider, whether in the form of written instructions which the patient takes with her or him to consult later when needed, scheduled follow-up visits or phone calls to check on whether the patient remembers and understands instructions can also influence both timing and correctness of use.

Relational

The relationship or setting within which a method is used can have an impact on effectiveness as well, both in terms of the knowledge the couple has about how to use the method and the ease at which it can be used. The type and stage of relationship can be important. Some women as well as men may be more apt or less apt to use a contraceptive with someone they do not know well or do not have a regular relationship with (Kisker, 1985). In general, the early stages of relationships are the riskiest times for unintended pregnancy to occur.

The degree of communication with one's partner as well as the partner's cooperation, knowledge and opinions can affect how easy it is to use a method. These factors are most relevant to the coitus related methods of condom, diaphragm, spermicides and periodic abstinence. With the exception of the diaphragm which can be inserted well in advance of intercourse, these other methods all require use at or near the time of intercourse and involve the knowledge and cooperation of both partners. While two partners can increase the amount of knowledge and commitment to method use, they can also confuse each other or exert pressure against consistent, accurate use.

Personal

Factors related to contraceptive use effectiveness that have been most often studied are personal characteristics. These influence whether a method is used at all and what method is chosen. Among method users, they influence both the timing and the correctness of use. Many of them are thought not to have an impact in and of themselves, but to serve as indicators for unmeasured variables such as motivation, skill and resources, as well as fecundity and frequency of intercourse.

Among the sociodemographic variables that have been investigated are age, parity, residence, education and pregnancy intentions. Variables such as these are usually readily available from sample surveys that include the contraceptive histories necessary for estimating rates of use effectiveness. Psychological factors found or posited to influence use effectiveness are internal versus external locus of control, fear of side effects from method use and the relative values placed on intercourse and pregnancy.

50

Economic factors, such as income and insurance coverage, can influence use effectiveness through the resources available to obtain contraceptive services as well as serve as proxies for other variables. The variations across subgroups and between countries in levels of use effectiveness suggest that there are cultural factors of importance as well. These might include norms regarding contraceptive usage, differences in strength of desire for number and spacing of children and the level of availability of contraceptive services and abortion services within the country. In addition to factors specifically related to contraceptive use and fertility behavior, countries also differ in attitudes about the use of medication, with different preferences and expectations regarding oral versus injectable medication, for example.

RESEARCH NEEDS

What has been presented here is primarily a framework for understanding and investigating factors affecting use effectiveness. It is grounded in logic, existing research and clinical reports and speculations. In fact, most work in this area has focused on measuring use effectiveness of methods and exploring the effects of personal, sociodemographic factors. Much more research is needed before there is adequate understanding of what factors are most relevant and how they operate.

We need:

· More information on what type of person is more apt to have contraceptive failure with each specific method.

· More information on why contraceptive failures occur.

· Better knowledge of how to help users be more effective.

ISSUES AND QUESTIONS

Even at the current state of knowledge about factors affecting contraceptive use effectiveness, some important questions exist.

First, is there a level of use effectiveness below which a method should not be made available as a contraceptive at all or for specific subgroups? While differences in effectiveness between mono-, bi-, and tri-phasic pill formulations may exist, they are so small as to be irrelevant for almost all groups of users. In contrast, introduction of new over-the-counter methods with relatively low levels of use effectiveness may well be inappropriate.

Second, how should data on effectiveness of contraceptives be presented to the public and to potential users? Slanted presentation or lack of full information can lead people to believe that methods are more effective than they are or less effective than data show to be the case. In both instances, people's choice of method and perhaps their pattern of use may be influenced by their incorrect perception of effectiveness.

It is clear, however, that unintended pregancies do occur among users of all types of contraceptives. The factors influencing the risk of contraceptive failure are complex and involve both the method itself and the person and couple using it. As a result, a pregnancy resulting from contraceptive failure should spur examination of why and how the pregnancy occurred, including review of method choice and how the method was used.

It is also clear that a pregnancy resulting from contraceptive failure is not always the woman's fault. Once it has occurred, the proper response is not to blame or punish the woman, but to help the woman deal with how best to resolve the pregnancy and how to lower her risk of experiencing another unintended pregnancy.

REFERENCES

Burnhill, M. Intrauterine contraception. In S. Corson, R. Derman, L. Tyrer, eds., Fertility Control. Little, Brown and Company, Boston, 1985.

Fraser, I. S., Jansen, R. P. Why do inadvertent pregnancies occur in oral contraceptive users? Effectiveness of oral contraceptive regimens and interfering factors. Contraception 27:531, 1983.

Johnson, V., Masters, W., K. C. Lewis. The physiology of intravaginal contraceptive failure. In M. S. Calderone, ed., Manual of Family Planning and Contraceptive Practice. Williams & Wilkins, Baltimore, Maryland, 1970.

Grady, W. R., Hirsch, M. B., Keen, N., Vaughan, B. Contraceptive failure and continuation among married women in the United States, 1970–1975. Studies in Family Planning 14:9, 1983.

Keith, L. F., Berger, G. S., Jackson, M. A. Foams, creams, and suppositories. In S. Corson, R. Derman, L. Tyler, eds., Fertility Control. Little, Brown and Company, Boston, Massachusetts, 1985.

Ketting, E., Leseman, P. Abortus en anticonceptie 1983/84. Stimezo-onderzoek, 1986.

Kisker, E. E. Teenagers talk about sex, pregnancy and contraception. Family Planning Perspectives 17:83, 1985.

Korteling, W., Cantel, S. "Dutch study confirms monophasic as most reliable pill." News and Views, published by Organon International at the Third Annual Meeting of The Society for the Advancement of Contraception in Bordeaux, France, September 1985.

Liskin, L., Fox, G. IUDs: an appropriate contraceptive for many women. Population Reports Series B, No. 4, 1982.

Orme, M. L., Back, D. F., Breckenridge, A. M. Drug interactions with oral contraceptive steroids. British Journal of Family Planning 10:19, 1984.

Orr, M. T. Private physicians and the provision of contraceptives to adolescents. Family Planning Perspectives 16:83, 1984.

Orr, M. T., Forrest, J. D. The availability of reproductive health services from U.S. private physicians. Family Planning Perspectives 17:63, 1985.

Pearl, R. Contraception and fertility in 2,000 women. Human Biology iv:363, 1932.

Potter, R. G. Application of life table technique to measurement of contraceptive effectiveness. Demography iii:297, 1966.

Tietze, C., Lewit, S. Statistical evaluation of contraceptive methods: Use-effectiveness and extended use-effectiveness. Demography 5:931, 1968.

Schirm, A. L., Trussell, J., Menken, J., Grady, W. R. Contraceptive failure in the United States: The impact of social, economic and demographic factors. Family Planning Perspectives 15:68, 1982.

Simon, P., Hakkou, F., Warot, D. Influence de certains medicaments sur les differents procedes de contraception. Contraception, Fertilite, Sexualite 12:479, 1984.

Soderstrom, R. Sterilization failures and their causes. Unpublished, 1984.

Vessey, M., Lawless, M., Yeates, D. Efficacy of different contraceptive methods. Lancet 1:841, 1982.

Wiley, A. T. The diaphragm. In S. Corson, R. Derman, L. Tyrer, eds., Fertility Control. Little, Brown and Company, Boston, Massachusetts, 1985.

ILLEGAL ABORTION AND EFFECT ON MEDICAL PRACTICE

AND PUBLIC HEALTH--NIGERIA

O. A. Ladipo

Professor of Obstetrics and Gynecology
College of Medicine
University College Hospital
Ibadan, Nigeria

INTRODUCTION

Although abortion laws have been liberalized in many countries, a restrictive abortion law still exists in Nigeria as well as in other countries in the Sub-Saharan region. In contemporary Nigeria the alarming increase in unwanted and unplanned pregnancy is of obvious concern to parents, policy makers, and government. However, there is an obvious reluctance on the part of government to initiate a liberal abortion law because of profound resentment from elders, religious leaders, and communities who have a strong pronatalist tradition. Despite these views and restrictive laws, illegal abortion is performed daily by skilled and unskilled persons who employ aseptic techniques and unorthodox methods with consequent high mortality and morbidity. While it is difficult to obtain national data on illegal abortion, hospital records on emergency admissions indicate that complications of abortion account for over 50 percent of the cases.

Since hospital records represent only the tip of the iceberg, the numbers of complicated induced abortion suggest an unmet need for contraceptive service and education. Nigeria, like most other African countries with restrictive laws, is currently at a stage of demographic transition where unwanted pregnancy and illegal abortion is high and access to contraceptive information and services is limited.

LEGAL STATUS OF INDUCED ABORTION

Among the countries of the world, the legal status of induced abortion ranges from complete prohibition to elective abortion at the request of the pregnant woman. A major consideration advanced by advocates of less restrictive abortion legislation, and especially of abortion on request, has been the benefit to public health. In those countries with restrictive abortion laws, poor and high parity women and unmarried adolescents represent the majority of women who seek illegal abortion, often resulting in compromised reproductive capacity or death. It is not surprising that the Nigerian "Termination of Pregnancy Bill" 1981, presented before the National Assembly, generated a lot of public interest and debate.

Many individuals felt that the traditional law is too strict and welcomed the effort at liberalization. Others felt that such liberalization would lead to even more sexual permissiveness and promiscuity in an already morally lax society. Some objected strongly on religious grounds. Unfortunately, the "Termination of

Pregnancy Bill" was aborted at its first reading without any parliamentary debate on the subject.

Present Nigerian Law regards as criminal any interference with pregnancy, however early it may take place except for therapeutic reasons as prescribed by the criminal and penal codes. The fetus is considered a human life to be protected by the criminal law from the moment of fertilization.

The relevant provisions of the Criminal Code applicable to the Southern States of Nigeria are stated in Sections 228 and 229 therein. It provides:

Any person who with intent to procure the miscarriage of a woman whether she is or not with child, unlawfully administers to her or causes her to take any poison or other noxious thing, or uses force of any kind, or uses any other means whatever is guilty of a felony. . . . Any woman who with intent to procure her own miscarriage, whether she is or not with child unlawfully adminsters to herself any poison or other noxious thing or uses force of any kind or uses other means to be administered or used by her is guilty of felony. . . .

Preservation of the mother's life is the only circumstance under the present law in which an abortion would be lawful--see Section 297 of the Code which states thus:

A person is NOT criminally responsible for performing in good faith and with reasonable care and skill a surgical operation . . . upon an unborn child for the preservation of the mother's life, if the performance of the operation is reasonable having regard to the patient's state at the time and all the circumstances of the case.

Similarly the Penal Code which applies to the Northern States of Nigeria provides in its Section 232 that:

Whoever voluntarily causes a woman with child to miscarry shall, if such miscarriage be not caused in good faith for the purpose of saving the life of the woman, be punished. . . .

CASE FOR ABORTION

Having stated the relevant provisions of the law as applicable in this country, it becomes necessary to set down the case usually made in favor of changing the abortion law and what direction that change should take.

The abortion debate is generally divided into two extreme views: those who regard abortion as virtually always evil and advocate a restrictive abortion policy, and those who regard abortion as entirely innocent and thus advocate a permissive policy. The latter is a liberal view chiefly advanced by the women's movement although one need not be a feminist to espouse it. The worst possible laws on abortion are those which are highly restrictive. Prohibiting abortion does not promote celibacy nor does liberalizing abortion promote promiscuity. The choice then for society is not between "abortion" or "no abortion." It is between abortion in safe, aseptic surroundings performed by qualified practitioners under the control and supervision of the law and abortion in filthy back-rooms performed by unscrupulous operators who are discovered and brought to justice only after the operation irrevocably and tragically has gone wrong.

Abortions can affect the birth rate, the medical practice and time allocations of doctors, the availability of hospital beds, the health and freedom of women, the use and effective use of contraceptives. The proper control of fertility should be by contraception and not by abortion, as repeat abortion may have a damaging effect both physically and psychologically. Private acts with ascertainable public consequences become a matter of legitimate concern to the public and a legitimate subject for legislation. Thus, as long as induced abortions have any consequences for society, for family life and for the practice of medicine, society has the right to take a legal interest in them.

THE BILL

The Termination of Pregnancy Bill, while suffering from exceedingly unskillful drafting, did attempt to introduce into the law some useful abortion reforms. However, the title of the Bill is a misnomer, perhaps because of a desire to avoid the unsavoury connotations of the word "abortion."

It could have been more appropriately entitled the Abortion Law Reform Bill, which might have helped to bring to public awareness that we do have an abortion law in need of reform. Section 1(1) of the bill provides that:

It shall be lawful and legal when a pregnancy is terminated by a registered medical practitioner if two registered practitioners are of the opinion formed in good faith

(a) that the continuance of the pregnancy would involve risk to the life of a pregnant woman or of injury to the physical or mental health of the pregnant woman or any existing children of her family greater than if the pregnancy were terminated; or

(b) that there is substantial risk that if the child were born it would suffer such physical or mental abnormations as to be seriously handicapped.

While the rejected bill is criticized both for its inelegant drafting and for some of its provisions it is hoped that every effort will be made to re-introduce the bill with certain amendments although it may now take the form of a Decree.

ATTITUDE TOWARDS SEXUAL RELATIONS, CONTRACEPTION AND ABORTION

In view of the current restrictive abortion laws, and the rather sensitive nature of sexual behavior and contraception, there is likely to be considerable underreporting in survey research conducted on attitudes towards sexual relations, contraception, and abortion. Nevertheless, available data from community and hospital studies show some pertinent trends. Earlier reports from Togo, Nigeria, Sierra Leone, and Ghana (Acsadi, 1976; Caldwell, 1974; Caldwell and Igun, 1970; Harrell-Bond, 1975; Kumekpor, 1970) indicate that less than 5 percent of the women admitted having had induced abortions although a considerably higher percentage of the respondents in most studies acknowledged knowing about traditional and modern methods of induced abortion. For example, in 1969, 8,400 rural and urban men and women in Nigeria were surveyed. Only 2 percent of the men reported that their partners had undergone induced abortions, and only 1.3 percent of the women admitted having induced abortions. By contrast, 24 percent of the women and 38 percent of the men said they knew about modern and traditional abortion methods (Caldwell and Igun, 1970).

Unwanted pregnancy and illegal abortion are subjects of concern in Nigeria. Limited existing data, most frequently obtained from hospital records, suggest that sexual activity among unmarried adolescents, particularly in urban areas, is increasing. Of significance too is the high percentage of adolescents in documented cases of illegal abortion (Akingba and Gbajumo, 1969). A review of hospital records from University of Benin Teaching Hospital between January 1, 1974, to December 31, 1979, revealed that approximately 71.7 percent of induced abortion occurred among primary and secondary school students. Only 9.8 percent were married. In an earlier study by Akingba and Gbajumo (1969), 60.8 percent of the patients were adolescent girls and 53.7 percent of them had had septic abortion. 91.2 percent of the study population was unmarried. Oronsaye and Odiase (1983), who reported on attitudes towards abortion and contraception among secondary school girls in Benin City, Nigeria, revealed that 21.1 percent of respondents had their first sexual experience before the age of 15 years while 30.2 percent of 530 respondents admitted to having had illegally induced abortion. Among the abortion group, 81.2 percent were single teenage girls aged 15—19. In general, the study group had a negative attitude to formal contraception. Only 6 percent ever used the "pill," while 44 percent had never used any contraceptive method.

A study on sexual behavior, contraceptive practice and reproductive health among the young unmarried population in Ibadan, Nigeria, aged 14—25 (Ladipo, et al., 1984) was conducted between November 1981 to March 1982. The sample was largely purposive, self-selected, and voluntary, and consisted of four distinct subgroups defined largely by age and education. Nine hundred fifty-nine of respondents were males while 841 were females. Eighty-one percent of all male respondents and 69 percent of female respondents approved of sexual relations before marriage, particularly among couples who are engaged to be married. Interestingly, only 66 percent of males contrasted with 78 percent of females also approved of the use of contraception. Sexual activity among the respondents varied from 38 percent of female secondary students to 90 percent among working-class males. The mean age for initial sexual experience was 16 years. Among all 18 year olds, 51 percent of the women and 78 percent of the men had engaged in sexual intercourse.

Of the sexually active adolescents, the better educated reported contraceptive use more frequently. Overall, 48 percent of sexually active males and 66 percent of sexually active females had used contraception at some time. Non-users overwhelmingly cited lack of knowledge about contraception as the main reason for not using any method, followed by concern over the safety of modern contraception. Consequently, it is not surprising that a high proportion of female respondents had experienced a pregnancy. Of all sexually active females, 45 percent reported having had at least one pregnancy rising to 62 percent among working class females.

One hundred eighty-three of 203 first pregnancies were interrupted by means of induced abortion. This figure, however, reflects some degree of self-selection, since in-school samples exclude women who became pregnant and elected to carry the pregnancy to term.

Despite the illegality of abortion in Nigeria, between one-fourth and one-half of the students surveyed said they would advise friends with unwanted pregnancies to opt for induced abortion. Over two-thirds of the working females would give such counsel, while only one-fourth of their male counterparts would do so. In an unpublished Monrovia Adolescent Study, 33 percent of a non-student community sample and 53 percent of a school sample reported terminating a pregnancy. In Oronsaye and Odiase's study (1983), only 15 percent of the control subjects and 50 percent of the abortion subjects considered abortion "wrong under any circumstances" (abortion is murder), while 58 percent and 55 percent of respondents respectively favored induced abortion on medical grounds.

RATIONALE FOR INDUCED ABORTION

The typical patient seeking induced abortion is young, unmarried, and in school. As many institutions dismiss pregnant school girls, the pregnant adolescent is likely to be forced to abandon her education unless some other solution is found (Akingba, 1972; Akinla, 1970; Bleek, 1977). In most studies on induced abortion in Africa, the desire to complete school training or remain gainfully employed and the fear of dismissal is the principal motivating rationale for seeking to terminate unplanned pregnancy. Sixty-eight percent of the cases of induced abortion surveyed by Akingba and Gbajumo (1969) cited fear of dismissal as the reason for adolescents in Lagos seeking clandestine abortion. Two-thirds of the adolescents surveyed by Oronsaye and Odiase (1983) cited similar reasons. Results from other West African studies concur (Ampofo, 1970; Ayangade, 1984).

Other less frequently cited reasons for induced abortion are economic constraints, taboo against illegitimate pregnancy, and pregnancy resulting from extramarital union.

Of interest as well is the tension caused by attitudes towards premarital sexuality and the premium set by Nigerian society on childbearing and parenthood. It is thought that many prospective bridegrooms demand proof of fertility from their fiancees or girlfriends as a prerequisite to marriage. Adolescents may thus feel obligated to establish their fertility through premarital conception despite lingering societal taboos on premarital sexuality. This explains in part why unwanted pregnancies among adolescents are on the increase and why illegal abortion is common despite Nigeria's restrictive abortion laws.

MEDICAL COMPLICATIONS OF ILLEGAL ABORTIONS

Illegal abortion with its myriad of complications is on the increase, in particular among adolescents. Mortality and morbidity from clandestine illegal abortion is still high in developing countries due to unskilled abortionists and the use of unhygenic facilities. Number of deaths from complications of abortion varies from 2.2 to 25.19 per 1,000 hospital admissions based on hospital reports from various parts of Africa (Akingba, 1977; Ampofo, 1973; Lwanga, 1977; Mati, 1977; Oronsaye, 1984). As much as 50 percent of all maternal deaths are the result of complications of illegal adolescent abortions in Nigeria (Akingba, 1972; Ojo, 1978). In a 1970 Study in Lagos, 11 percent of all teenage women hospitalized with complications from induced abortion died (Akingba and Gbajumo, 1969). Morbidity of illegal abortion is more difficult to measure although more common. Perhaps the most frequent complication of illegal abortion is incomplete evacuation with a variety of complications.

Septic abortions constitute a special problem in our gynaecological practice and indeed are the most common life-threatening complication and the most common cause of death from induced abortion, whether legal or illegal. The clinical picture is often that of a young unmarried school girl presenting with fever, abdominal pain, and foul-smelling blood-stained vaginal discharge. She is usually moribund, apprehensive, and toxic. Some of these patients present in terminal stages of septicemic shock with varying degrees of hepato-renal failure, jaundice, and occasionally severe bleeding due to disseminated intravascular coagulopathy. A few cases may be psychotic, restless, have flight of ideas, and exhibit grandiose delusion. The majority of these patients die because of inadequate facilities for investigations and management. Appropriate chemotherapy is usually limited and too expensive for the average client. The few that survive septic abortion subsequently suffer chronic pelvic inflammatory disease with periodic acute exarcerbation, congestive dysmenorrhea, dyspareunia. This often leads to indiscriminate use of antibiotics and analgesic drugs at great cost, with varying degrees of symptomatic relief. In any culture, in particular in the African society, the long-term effect of septic abortion resulting in compromised reproductive potential has serious social, economic, and psychological implications in view of the very high premium placed on childbearing and parenthood.

When illegal abortion is procured by instrumentation, trauma to the genital tract is often accompanied by visible and concealed hemorrhage leading to hypovolumic shock and pallor. Perforation of the uterus with a damaged viscus needs urgent exploratory laparotomy, while a torn cervix needs to be skillfully repaired. Often, over-enthusiastic cervical dilatation during repeated midtrimester abortion results in subsequent cervical incompetence with future reproductive failure. Subsequent poor reproductive performance often leads to regrets, remorse, marital disharmony, depression, and ultimately divorce or separation.

Literature reviews indicate that women who have had repeated induced abortions may run an increased risk of subsequent adverse reproductive outcome. The possibility of higher risk of miscarriage, prematurity, and low birth weight previously reported were critically reviewed by Cates (1981). He concluded that there was no demonstrable consistency whether repeat abortion per se produces increased risk of adverse reproductive outcome in subsequent desired pregnancies. Rather, his review suggested that technical subtleties of the abortion procedure affected the outcomes of published investigations most, while uncontrolled differences in patient characteristics could have explained in part the conflicting results among the studies.

Complications vary from country to country depending to a large extent on the skill of the abortionist, facilities for inducing abortion, and gestational age. In general, where abortion is legalized, the safest effective technology is used and necessary safety precautions are observed. In most countries with restrictive laws, the client's only option is the clandestine practitioner who charges exorbitant fees and has little consideration for the safety of the client. In a recent publication from University of Benin Teaching Hospital, Benin City, Nigeria, 90 percent of abortionists involved in cases of admitted induced abortions were quacks or charlatans (Oronsaye, 1984).

Noteworthy is the considerable drain on limited hospital resources by patients admitted for complications of induced abortion. The majority of the cases who survive the first 48 hours of admission occupy hospital beds for 2–8 weeks (Akingba and Gbajumo, 1969; Oronsaye, 1984) depending on the nature of their complications. The cost of treatment in terms of chemotherapy, blood transfusion, and operative management is staggering. In many developing countries, only a few hospitals are adequately equipped to cope with complicated cases of illegal abortion, in particular those that are associated with severe sepsis and hemorrhage, hence the high mortality associated with illegal abortion.

INDUCED ABORTION AND CONTRACEPTION

The observed global change in sexual behavior, in particular among the young, is to a large extent responsible for the increased prevalence of unwanted pregnancy. In most African countries with restrictive abortion laws, the breakdown of traditional norms that regulated sexual behavior led to staggering levels of unwanted pregnancy. These are usually terminated illegally despite the risk of death. Most of these countries also have a strong pronatalist posture which discourages contraceptive usage for preventive purpose or termination of fertility.

Most developing countries are currently at a stage of demographic transition where family size is limited by induced abortion rather than use of effective modern contraception. Experience from the University College Hospital, Ibadan, indicates that women who have had an abortion are more highly motivated than other women to use an effective method of contraception (Ladipo and Ojo, 1978). Other studies have also shown that for most women the abortion experience has led to enhanced knowledge and practice of contraception (Akhter and Rider, 1984; Potts et al., 1977; Bhatia and Ruzicka, 1980; Margolis et al., 1974). The relationship between abortion and contraception is complementary rather than competitive. Induced abortion offers the opportunity for contraceptive education and counseling which should be optimized by physicians.

In a recently concluded study in Ibadan, Nigeria, the dynamics of the pituitary hormone (luteinizing hormone, follicular-stimulating hormone, prolactin) and progesterone in normal, adult Nigerian females during their first post abortal cycle, indicate that 82 percent attained LH peak within the first 22 days after menstrual regulation. This finding underlines the importance of stressing the need for contraceptive counseling during this vulnerable period (Osotimehin et al., 1984).

CONCLUSION

Induced abortion, the oldest method of human birth control, remains the major cause of maternal mortality and morbidity in Africa. Despite restrictive abortion laws, the incidence of abortion is escalating because of lack of effective contraceptive knowledge and services, preference for smaller families, desire for higher education, increase in the number of women of childbearing age and the current economic crisis. Women seeking abortion are demonstrating an intense desire to avoid unwanted births. A priority of governments with restrictive abortion laws must be to recognize the adverse complications associated with illegal abortion and to formulate rational policies that would accelerate reproductive health education and encourage the use of modern contraceptives. A more liberal policy on abortion would also considerably reduce the currently high mortality and morbidity associated with illegal abortion.

For any woman, illegal abortion is physically and psychologically traumatic with immediate risk to life, health, and future fertility. Undoubtedly, most women are ignorant of the varied risks, while enlightened others would rather accept these risks in a desperate attempt to avoid illegitimate birth. For an individual, the risks and costs are high. For the community, illegal abortion incur both human and financial costs by imposing a heavy burden on limited health care resources.

ACKNOWLEDGMENT

This is to express my profound gratitude to the International Women's Health Coalition for inviting me to participate in the "Christopher Tietze International Symposium." Their global contribution to the improvement of reproductive health is unique and highly commendable. I also thank Mr. Adyanju for secretarial assistance.

REFERENCES

Acsadi, G. T. Traditional birth control methods in Yorubaland. In J. F. Marshall, S. Polgar, eds., Culture, Natality and Family Planning. Caroline Population Centre (Monograph 21 p. 126), 1976.

Akhter, H. N., Rider, R. V. Menstrual regulation and contraception in Bangladesh: Competing or Complementary. International Journal of Gynaecology and Obstetrics 22:137, 1984.

Akingba, J. B., Gbajuma, S. A. Procured abortion--counting the cost, Journal of the Nigerian Medical Association 6:16, 1969.

Akingba, J. B. The Problem of Unwanted Pregnancies in Nigeria Today. Nigeria University of Lagos Press, Lagos, 1972.

Akingba, J. B. Abortion, maternity and other health problems in Nigeria. Nigerian Medical Journal 7(4):465, 1977.

Akinla, O., Adadevoh, B. K. Abortion a medico-social problem. Journal of the Nigerian Medical Association 6:16, 1969.

Akinla, O. Abortion in Africa. In R. E. Hall, ed., Abortion in a Changing World. Vol 1 (Proceedings of the 6th World Congress on Fertility and Sterility, Tel Aviv. May 20–27, 1968), p. 113. Israel Academy of Sciences and Humanities, Jerusalem, 1970.

Ampofo, D. A. The dynamics of induced abortion and the social implication for Ghana. Ghana Medical Journal 9:295, 1970.

Ampofo, D. A. Epidemiology of abortion in selected African countries. Presented at the IPPF Conference on the Medical and Social Aspects of Abortion in Africa, p. 22, Accra, Ghana, Dec. 12–18, 1973.

Ayangade, S. O. Contraceptive knowledge and practice among induced abortion patients, Nigerian experience. Paper presented at the International Symposium on Reproductive Health Care, Maui, Oct. 10–15, 1982. Abstract in Contraceptive Delivery Systems 3.419, 1984.

Bhatia, S., Ruzicka, L. T. Menstrual regulation clients in a village based family planning programme. Journal of Biosocial Science 12:31, 1980.

Bleek, W. Family planning of birth control, the Ghananian contradiction. Cultures et Development 9(i):64, 1977.

Caldwell, J. C. The study of fertility and fertility change in tropical Africa, Voorburg, Netherlands International Statistical Institute. World Fertility Survey Occasional Papers 7:35, May 1974.

Caldwell, J. C., Igun, A. The spread of anti-natal knowledge and practice in Nigeria. Population Studies 24(1):21, 1970.

Cates, W., Jr. Repeat induced abortions, do they affect future childbearing. Presented at 37th Annual Meeting of the American Fertility Society, Atlanta, Georgia, March 1981.

Harrell-Bond, B. Some influential attitudes about family limitation and the use of contraceptives among the professional group in Sierra-Leone. In J. C. Caldwell, ed., Population Growth and Socioeconomic Change in West Africa, pp. 473. Columbia University Press, New York, 1975.

Kumekpor, T. K. Rural women and attitudes to family planning, contraceptive practice and abortion in Southern Togo. Socio-demographic Study of the Republic of Togo 1:30, 1970.

Ladipo, O. A., Nichols, D. J., Delano, G. E., Otolorin, E. O. Reproductive health attitudes and practices--Nigeria. Pathpapers 11:10, 1984.

Ladipo, O. A., Ojo, O. A. Menstrual regulation in Ibadan, Nigeria. International Journal of Gynaecology and Obstetrics 15:428, 1978.

Lwanga, C. Abortion in Mulago Hospital, Kampala. East African Medical Journal 53(3):142, 1977.

Margolis, A., Rindfuss, R., Coughlar, P., Rochat, R. Contraception and abortion. Family Planning Perspectives 6:56, 1974.

Mati, J. K. H. Abortion in Africa. In F. T. Sai, ed., Family Welfare and Development in Africa, p. 74. IPPF, London, 1977.

Ojo, O. A. Septic abortion in Ibadan, a ten year review of cases. West Africa Medical Journal 26:51, 1978.

Okojie, S. E. Induced illegal abortion in Benin City, Nigeria. International Journal of Gynaecology and Obstetrics 14:517, 1976.

Oronsaye, A. U., Odiase, G. I. Attitudes towards abortion and contraception among Nigerian secondary school girls. International Journal of Gynaecology and Obstetrics 21:423, 1983.

Oronsaye, A. U. Maternal mortality due to abortions at UBTH, Benin City. Tropical Journal of Obstetrics and Gynaecology 5.1:23, 1984.

Osotimehin, B., Otolorin, E. O., Ladipo, O. A. Sequential Hormone Measurements after First Trimester Abortion in Normal Nigerian Women, 1984. In press.

Ovin, A. E., Oronsaye, A. U., Fall, M. K. B., et al. Adolescent induced abortion in Benin City, Nigeria. International Journal of Gynaecology and Obstetrics 19:495, 1981.

Potts, M., Diggory, P., Peel, J. Abortion. Cambridge University Press, Cambridge, 1977.

UTILIZATION OF INDUCED ABORTION IN KOREA

Sung-bong Hong

Chairman
Department of Obstetrics and Gynecology
Korea University Hospital
Seoul, Korea

Compared to other developing countries in Asia, Korea is known to be one of the countries where population growth was fairly well reduced within a short period of time.

A major contributing factor in reducing such population growth is attributable to induced abortion which is now legal only in limited cases on medical and philanthropic grounds. But in practice the abortion rate surpassed even the levels of those countries where abortions are legalized without limitation.

LEGAL STATUS OF INDUCED ABORTION

Officially, the penal code against induced abortion is still effective. However, actual judicial supervision has become nominal with the growing emphasis on population control. Since the launch of the government programs in family planning in the early 1960s, demands for abortion have shifted gradually from urban to rural areas. At the same time, the medical profession came to play a role as service providers.

Belatedly the Maternal and Child Health Law (Hong, 1974) enacted in January 1973, as shown in Table 1 permitted a physician to perform an abortion with the consent of the woman and her spouse only in case of familial hereditary disease, certain infectious diseases, when the pregnancy resulted from rape or incest, or when the continuation of pregnancy would severely compromise maternal health. Socio-economic grounds were not included.

In reality, however, the actual practice of induced abortion had been liberalized even long before the enactment of the law. The government has attempted to legalize abortion to the full extent, including socioeconomic grounds, several times in order to solve the inconsistency between legal status and actual practice, but failed due to persistent protest from religious sectors.

PREVALENCE OF INDUCED ABORTION AND ITS NEW TREND

Due to the lack of a good reporting system of induced abortion, data produced from the sampling surveys are indispensable for the estimation of induced abortions. Fortunately, a considerable amount of the survey data on induced abor-

Table 1: Maternal and Child Health Law

Article 8. Indication for Abortion

1. When suffering from eugenic and hereditary mental and physical disease.

2. When the person herself suffers from infectious diseases designated by a presidential decree.

3. When pregnancy results from rape or incest.

4. When pregnancy results from intermarriage which is prohibited by law.

5. When the continuation of pregnancy is extremely detrimental to the health of the mother.

---

tion have been accumulated since the 1960s. The prevalence rate (Hong, 1976; Byun, 1979; Lim, 1982) of induced abortions among married women in Seoul was 25 percent in 1964; doubled to 50 percent in 1976, and rose to 58 percent in 1978. In rural areas the prevalence was only 4 percent in 1964, 19 percent in 1971, and rose to 38 percent in 1978. As to the national rate, it was 7 percent in 1964, 26 percent in 1971, and rose to 49 percent in 1978. In 1982, about one half of married women reportedly had experienced induced abortion (49.6 percent).

The main reason listed for induced abortion in these married Korean women was to control family size. Thus, the highest abortion rate is to be expected among the age group whose family building is about to be completed. The highest rate has been in age 30–34 except for the data in 1978, where the highest rate was in the 25–29 age group. The age of married women seeking abortion has been shifting from their thirties to late twenties in the last two decades; age-specific abortion rate for married women in their 20s increased by five times, tripled for those in their 30s, and doubled for those in their 40s (Hong, 1979). Furthermore, an abortion provider's survey in 1979 in Seoul disclosed that nulliparous women comprised 46.6 percent of all abortions, women in their early twenties represented about 40 percent, and those in their late twenties 25 percent of the total abortions. Thus, women in their twenties comprised two-thirds (65.2 percent) of all women undergoing abortions in Seoul.

The proportion of unmarried women having abortions is estimated in the range of 28.7 to 38.5 percent. This changing age pattern of aborters in recent years implies that abortion was used for the limitation of family size in the 1960s, and in the 1970s it is sought by younger adults for fertility control.

CIRCUMSTANCES SURROUNDING THE PRACTICE OF INDUCED ABORTION

Facilities

According to a national survey in 1971 (Hong, 1976), the majority (84 percent) of induced abortions in Korea are performed at the clinics of private physicians (Table 2). The proportion is higher in Seoul (90 percent) than in rural areas (81 percent). General hospitals are the site for only 7 percent of abortions and the remaining 9 percent are performed in other medical facilities. In Seoul, 4 percent of abortions are performed in nonmedical facilities, but this proportion rises to 12 percent in rural areas in 1971. Economic improvement coupled with the

Table 2: Percent Distribution of Place of Performance, 1971

Place of Performance	All Korea	Seoul	Other Urban	Rural
Private Clinic	84	90	83	81
General Hospital	7	6	8	7
Non-medical facilities	9	4	9	12
Sample size (N)	1,289	356	380	553

increasing coverage of medical insurance in recent years, makes it more likely that almost all aborters are utilizing medical facilities.

Methods

A survey of providers (Hong, 1979) of abortion services in Seoul during 1977–1978 showed that 30 percent used surgical curettage and 9 percent suction curettage exclusively, while 61 percent used combined methods for abortion in the first trimester (Table 3). Surgical curettage was almost always performed under general anesthesia.

About 15 percent of the providers using suction curettage did so under local anesthesia. One in three performed very early suction procedures, using a flexible cannula with a diameter of 4–6mm, without anesthesia. This very early suction procedure has been subsidized by the government for limited numbers of abortions (about 20,000 cases per year) when the pregnancy resulted from IUD failure, or surgical sterilization.

For midtrimester abortion the preferred methods were metreurynter (intra-uterine balloon), intravenous infusion of oxytocics, and insertion of bougies or laminaria tents. Few providers used intra- or extra-amniotic instillations of either hypertonic saline or prostaglandin and even fewer reported hysterotomy or instrumental evacuation by the vaginal route.

Agents

As Table 4 indicates, more than 90 percent of Korean abortions had been performed by physicians, one-half (48.8 percent) by specialists in obstetrics and gynecology, 14.4 percent by surgeons, and 36.8 percent by general practitioners (Hong, 1979). In 1971, 4 percent of the abortions were performed by nonphysicians in Seoul, 12 percent in rural areas. Thus women in rural areas had less access to a physician and much less access to a specialist.

COMPLICATIONS AND MORTALITY FOLLOWING ABORTIONS

Complications related to induced abortions are "always larger than zero" as Christopher Tietze described in his last edition of Induced Abortion--1983. It is difficult to ascertain complication rates in private clinics which have no official reporting system. However, since abortions are performed there mostly by physicians, the rate of complication is assumed to be relatively low despite the illegal status of abortion.

On the other hand there may be a few drawbacks in terms of medical safety at free-standing clinics. Abortions are often carried out by general practitioners.

Table 3: Methods of Termination of
Pregnancy in First Trimester

Methods	Percent
Surgical Curettage	30
Suction Curettage	9
Both Methods	61
	100

Table 4: Estimated Annual Number and Percent of Induced Abortion,
by Type of Providers, Seoul Korea, 1977/78

Item	Number of Induced Abortions	Percent
Total	533,000	100.0
Types of Providers		
Public hospital	14,000	2.6
Private hospital	13,000	2.5
Private clinic	506,000	94.9
Provider's Specialization		
OB/GYN	260,000	48.8
Surgeon	77,000	14.4
G.P.	196,000	36.8
Period of Gestation		
1st trimester	490,000	91.9
2nd trimester	36,000	6.8
3rd trimester	7,000	1.3

Table 5: Causes of Maternal Deaths Due to Induced Abortion in Seoul

Hospitals	Periods Covered	Infections	Hemorrhage	Others	Total	Total Maternal Deaths
Ewha University Hospital	'61–'76	4	2	--	6	90
Red Cross Hospital	'72–'77	2	1	--	3	64
Hankang Sacred Heart Hospital	'72–'78	7	2		9	41
National Medical Center	'66–'77	8	8	13	29	65
		21	13	13	47	260

In addition, abortions are permissable up to 28 weeks of gestation when most of the grave complications may occur. The occurrence of sepsis and hemorrhage is presumably not rare at private clinics particularly where most of the mid-trimester abortions occur, but there are no data on the frequency of such occurrences.

Data on mortality, even though the event is obvious, are fragmentary and inconclusive.

Reports from several general hospitals in Seoul (Table 5) disclosed that the proportion of deaths due to induced abortion comprises 18 percent (47 cases) of a total of 260 maternal deaths collected from four hospitals covering different lengths of time periods, with about 4.5 deaths per year on pooled samples. A fair estimate for deaths in Seoul alone would be somewhere between 20 and 30 per year covering a total of about 500,000 abortions per year.

IMPACT OF ILLEGAL ABORTION ON THE HEALTH OF WOMEN

As previously mentioned, induced abortion in Korea is theoretically illegal if it is performed for socio-economic reasons. However, in reality, almost all abortions are undertaken by qualified physicians. Accordingly, the legal status of induced abortion appears to have no direct bearing on the health of women.

Several aspects from the medical viewpoint seem worthy to note. Abortion in the mid-trimester, which is often with poor outcome, still comprises about 8 percent of all procedures (Table 4). In addition, fatal cases due to sepsis or hemorrhage are infrequently reported.

As to the late sequelae of induced abortion, the results of a prospective study conducted in Seoul under the auspices of the WHO, were insufficient to conclude any significance of association of induced abortion with subsequent sterility and ectopic pregnancy compared to first childbirth.

Concerns for the woman's health should consider the new trend that indicates an estimated annual induced abortion rate of about one and a half million. Of this number, one half will be nulliparous women in their early twenties.

REFERENCES

Byun, J. H., Koh, K. S. 1978 Family Planning and Fertility Survey. Korea Institute for Family Planning, 1979.
Hong, S. B. Induced Abortion (III). The New Medical Journal 17:43, 1974.
Hong, S. B., Watson, W. A. The Increasing Utilization of Induced Abortion in Korea. Korea University Press, Seoul, 1976.
Hong, S. B. Recent changes in patterns of induced abortion in Seoul. Korean Journal of Obstetrics and Gynecology 22:795, 1979.
Hong, S. B., Tietze, C. Survey of abortion providers in Seoul, Korea. Studies in Family Planning 10:161, 1979.
Lee, N. H., Lee, J. O. Maternal mortality, a 20 year study (1961–1980). Korean Journal of Obstetrics and Gynecology 25:12, 1982.
Lim, J. K. Current status of induced abortion. Journal of Population and Health Studies, Korean Institute for Population and Health 2:166, 1982.
Tietze, C. Induced Abortion: A World Review, 1983. Population Council, New York, 1983.

INDUCED ABORTION IN LATIN AMERICA: IMPACT ON HEALTH

Benjamin Viel

Professor of Preventive Medicine
Faculty of Medicine, University of Chile
Member, Academia de Medicina
Instituto de Chile
Santiago, Chile

Induced abortion on request is illegal in all Spanish- and Portuguese-speaking countries of Latin America, with Cuba, where abortion was legalized in 1979, the only exception.

In most of the Latin American countries, therapeutic abortion is permitted; in some if the continuation of the pregnancy endangers the woman's life, in others if it seriously threatens her physical health. In a few countries, induced abortion is also legal if the pregnancy is the consequence of rape or incest. In only three Latin American countries (Dominican Republic, Panama, and Haiti), induced abortion is illegal under all circumstances (Tietze, 1983).

Nontherapueutic abortion is punishable as a crime under the penal codes in all Latin American countries, except Cuba. The codes specify the severity of the prison terms for those who perform an illegal abortion, as well as for those who submit to it. I should like to emphasize, however, that the punishment for performing an illegal abortion as laid down in the penal codes is far less severe and the prison term is far shorter than the penalties exacted for taking the life of another human being. It follows, then, that in Latin American countries (except Cuba) abortion is a crime punishable under their penal codes, but it is not equivalent to murder and is, in terms of the penalties prescribed, a far lesser crime.

The principal effect of these restrictive measures is to make abortion more difficult to obtain and more dangerous for poor women. As for rich women who wish to terminate their pregnancy, there is no city on the Latin American continent where they cannot obtain an illegal abortion performed by an experienced and well-qualified professional. The cost is, of course, high, since the woman pays for the abortion as well as for the risk which the professional is taking. No records are kept of these procedures. Furthermore, since induced abortion today, if performed early in pregnancy, is medically safe and major complications requiring hospitalization are extremely rare, the number of voluntary induced abortions among the well-to-do sectors of our society is at present and will always remain unknown.

The situation is different for that large majority of women who are unable to pay the high cost of a medically safe abortion. A poor woman who has an unwanted pregnancy has only two options. She may go to an empirical abortionist or an unqualified practitioner for a cheap, clandestine procedure and face the risk of a major complication, or she may attempt a self-induced abortion with the high probability of a major complication which in a substantial proportion of the cases ends in death.

CHILE

Hospital records in Chile are good and 95 percent of all deliveries take place in hospitals. The records of the Census Bureau and the Civil Registration Service are also reliable. Nevertheless, I feel that the information from the hospital records of Santiago, the capital city, is more complete. I have therefore collected data on the number of women hospitalized in Santiago with the diagnosis of abortion for each year between 1940 and 1984. The data include both spontaneous and induced abortion, since it was impossible to distinguish them in the hospital records. On the basis of an estimate of the total number of women between 15 and 49 years of age, I computed the rate of hospitalization for abortion per thousand women of fertile age and compared it, by year, with the infant mortality rate per thousand live births. (See Figure 1.)

The figure shows that from 1940 to 1964 the infant mortality rate declined so rapidly that in 1964 it was one-half of the level it was in 1940. Mothers of Chilean families became aware that family size was no longer controlled by the early death of their children. Family size began to increase annually, while the resource for its support remained static.

Since no effective contraceptives were available prior to 1960, women resorted to induced abortion as the only way they knew to control the size of their families and to fulfill their responsibilities to the children already born. Between 1960 and 1964, physicians specializing in obstetrics and gynecology and in public health brought to the attention of the Ministry of Health that they were faced with a virtual epidemic of induced abortion. By 1964, hospitalizations for abortion in Santiago reached a peak of 48 per 1,000 women in reproductive age.

Several epidemiologic studies conducted in the early 1960s (Armijo and Monreal, 1964; Requena, 1969; Plaza and Briones, 1963) utilized the data available from hospital records, as I have done, supplementing these with carefully constructed questionnaire surveys conducted with representative samples of several

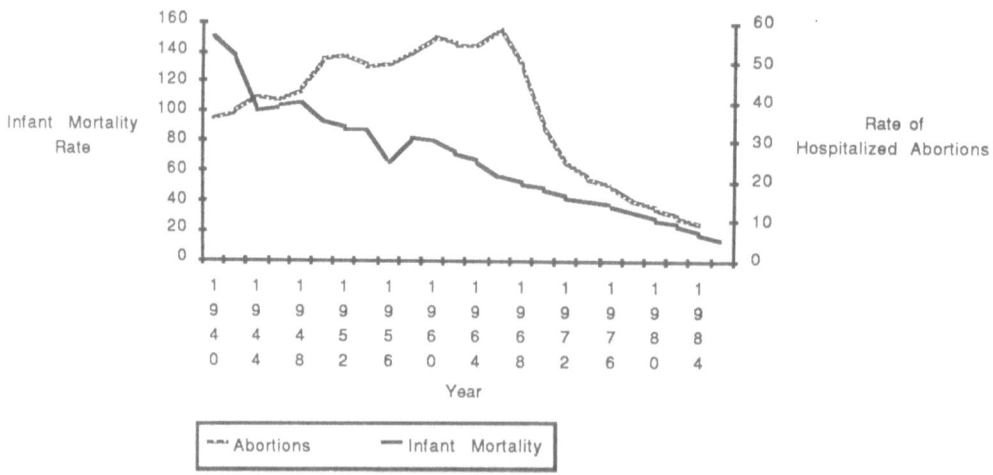

Fig. 1. Rates of Infant Mortality per 1,000 Live Births and Hospitalized Abortions per 1,000 Women of Fertile Age, Santiago, Chile, 1940–84.

communities to ascertain the retrospective frequency of induced abortion in Chile. On the basis of the data it was concluded that:

1. The frequency of induced abortion observed in Santiago was the same in all other urban areas in Chile, and was lower in rural areas.

2. Hospitalized cases of abortion were only the tip of the iceberg. For each hospitalized case there were two which did not require hospitalization.

3. Eighty percent of the women who reported having had an induced abortion were married or living in common-law unions, were 20 to 34 years of age (with a mean age of 27 years), and had two to four living children prior to the abortion. It appears, then, that induced abortion was used to limit the family size.

4. The great majority of those who had submitted to an induced abortion reported themselves as Catholics and the degree of religiosity appears to have had no influence on their decision to have an abortion.

5. Maternal mortality attributed to induced abortion in 1964 was close to one-half of maternal mortality for all causes.

6. Hospitalized abortion cases cost the Public Health sector of the country as a whole an estimated one million dollars.

7. The larger number of hospitalized beds occupied by women suffering from the complications of abortion created a shortage of beds for women with normal deliveries. Between 1960 and 1964, physicians tended to see two puerperal women per bed, discharging most of them within 24 hours of delivery. Thus, these normal puerperal women with their day-old infants had to go home to take care of other children at home, as well as attend to the usual housework, without a proper period of post-delivery rest. No doubt this situation was a contributing factor to high neonatal mortality observed at that time (40.2 per 1,000 born--Departamento de Estadistica del Servicio Nacional de Salud, 1965).

These findings convinced the Ministry of Health in Chile that an effective contraceptive was the only possible alternative to induced abortion. Furthermore, it was common knowledge that the restrictive abortion laws were not respected. Physicians did not report women who were hospitalized for incomplete abortions to the police. If they had, the already crowded jails would have been unable to accommodate the convicted women, much less their accomplices. Furthermore, no provision had been made for the care of the imprisoned women. All these obstacles prevented the implementation of the restrictive abortion laws.

Between 1960 and 1964 few clinics were offering effective contraceptives (IUDs and pills) but on a limited scale and only in major cities. Since 1964 the National Health Service of the Chilean Ministry of Health has offered free contraceptive services on a voluntary basis. Acceptance of these services has been increasing annually. Today, it is estimated that 22 percent of all women of fertile age in Chile use some form of contraception, with 80 percent using IUDs. These figures exclude those who buy contraceptives without prescriptions and those who are under private medical care.

The effect of the official policy on contraception, instituted in 1964, on hospitalization for abortion is shown in Figure 1. Not only has the rate of hospitalizations for abortion per 1,000 women of reproductive age declined dramatically between the years 1964 to 1984, but deaths from abortion in Santiago dropped to 0.14 per 1,000 women of reproductive age, compared with an estimated rate six times higher 20 years before.

Figure 1 also shows that the decline in infant mortality became more pronounced in the last two decades, compared with the preceding two decades. Some part of this decline may be attributed to a decrease in multiparity. It has been established that children born to the grand multiparae have higher rates of infant mortality than those born into smaller families (Cabrera, 1982). In 1969, 25 percent of the births in Chile were of the fifth or higher order. In 1979, the comparable figure was 10 percent.

These data show that the use of effective contraceptive methods tends to reduce the incidence of induced abortion.

OTHER LATIN AMERICAN COUNTRIES

Studies conducted by the Center of Latin American Demography in four major cities—Buenos Aires, Argentina; Bogota, Colombia; Panama, Panama; and Lima, Peru—(Gaslonde, 1975) show results similar to those in Chile and discussed in the preceding paragraphs. Hospitalizations for abortion declined but did not disappear in those areas where adequate contraceptive services were available. Only in Lima, where such services were poor, did the number of abortions continue to rise. Studies conducted in Colombia by ASCOFAME (Asociacion Colombiana de Facultades de Medicina) (1978), as well as in Mexico City (Ordonez, 1967), show very similar results, leading me to the inevitable conclusion that the number of illegal abortions, especially those highly dangerous, clandestine procedures resorted to by the poor, can be reduced but not eradicated by the use of effective contraception. Some preventable deaths continue to occur.

Of all the data available on mortality by cause, perhaps the most unreliable is the information on deaths associated with abortion. In the first place, only those women who die in hospitals from abortions are reported. Table 1 presents figures on abortion mortality per 10,000 live births for those countries for which these data were available (Pan American Health Organization/World Health Organization) (OPS/OMS). The data show that preventable deaths attributed to induced abortion still occurred in 1978. The lowest mortality was reported for Cuba, where voluntary abortion was legalized in 1979, but authorized by the government and implemented some years before its formal legalization. The highest mortality associated with abortion was reported for Paraguay where abortion is illegal and effective contraceptive methods are not officially sanctioned.

Table 1: Deaths Due to Abortion per 10,000 Live Births; Latin American Countries, 1977—1980

Country	Deaths Due to Abortion
Argentina	2.5
Chile	2.4
Colombia	2.6
Cuba	0.4
Ecuador	1.3
El Salvador	0.7
Guatemala	1.1
Mexico	0.7
Paraguay	7.0
Peru	1.3
Venezuela	1.3

Source: OPS/OMS, Conditions of Health in the Americas (1977—1980), Scientific Publication No. 427.

CUBA

I have heard from Dr. Alvarez-Lajonchere (1982), former Professor of Obstetrics and Gynecology in Havana, about a study made in Cuba prior to 1970 in which the cause of out-of-hospital deaths of women 15 to 49 years of age was carefully investigated. Interviews were conducted with the physician who last saw the patient, or members of the family as well as friends, in the event a doctor had not attended the patient. The study revealed that complications from induced abortions were at that time the leading cause of death among women of reproductive age. These findings prompted the government to legalize abortion on request during the first 12 weeks of pregnancy and for medical indications later in pregnancy. The Cuban law provides that the abortion must be carried out in clinics approved by the Ministry of Health and must be free of charge. Penalties are prescribed for physicians who charge for the procedure.

In my estimation, a similar study conducted in other countries in Latin America would also reveal a high mortality from abortion. I, myself, have seen certificates signed by physicians with "gynecological infection" entered as the cause of death. If the physician were to admit that abortion was the true cause of death, he would waste time in legal formalities.

ADOLESCENT PREGNANCY

Sexual activity among adolescents is on the rise in every Latin American country in which the problem has been studied. In 1970 in Chile, deliveries to unmarried teenagers (under 20 years of age) constituted 30 percent of all deliveries in that age group. In 1983, unmarried adolescents accounted for 53 percent of all deliveries among those under 20 years of age (Instituto Nacional de Estadisticas Chile, unpublished). Children born out of wedlock to adolescent mothers are fast becoming a universal health problem. Reliable information exists for Chile that babies born to unwed mothers have the highest proportion and most severe cases of malnutrition recorded for all children (Monckeberg and Ruimallo, 1982).

Adolescents in Latin America, especially those living in overcrowded slum areas, do not receive adequate information on contraception. Furthermore, it is difficult for them to go to a clinic and they do not have the money to buy pills at a pharmacy. At the time of delivery at the Maternity Hospital of the city of Temuco, 83 percent of unmarried adolescents declared that they did not want to become pregnant and that they did not have the money to pay even an unqualified practitioner (Diener and Viel, to be published). The only country in the continent in which the adolescent fertility rate is on the decline is Cuba (Population Reference Bureau, 1981).

The prevailing prejudices in Latin America are such that in some countries the World Fertility Study was not permitted to interview females under the age of 20. In Chile the World Fertility Survey was not permitted by the government.

LATIN AMERICA'S DEMOGRAPHIC PROBLEM

The Center of Latin American Demography estimated that in 1980 the total population living on the continent was 363 million and predicted that the figure would reach 552 million by the year 2000 (CELADE, 1983), an increase of 189 million people in only two decades. In Latin America the quality of life is deteriorating, as has been shown in studies conducted by UNICEF (United Nations Children's Fund) (1982), in several countries during the second half of the seventies. I believe that demographic pressure will bring about further deterioration in the quality of life. I also believe that this deterioration will force governments to liberalize the present abortion laws. Signs in some Latin American countries indicate that such a change is already on the way.

In conclusion, I whould like to add this thought. It is becoming increasingly difficult for me to accept the differentiation between therapeutic and voluntary abortion. According to the WHO (World Health Organization) definition, health is a state of "physical, mental, and social well-being and not only the absence of disease." If a pregnant woman wishes to terminate her pregnancy while in a state of physical well-being, is she also in a state of mental and social well-being? If the answer is "no," and following the universally accepted definition just quoted, all induced abortions should be classified as therapeutic if performed under the sanitary, safe conditions that prevail in modern medical practice today.

Such a formulation does not imply that abortion should replace contraception. Preventive medicine is always superior to curative medicine. If abortion is ever legalized in Latin America, it should always be accompanied by preventive measures to avoid repeat abortions.

I thank the organizers of this Symposium for the great honor accorded me to present this paper in remembrance of a great scholar, a great friend, and a great gentleman--Christopher Tietze.

REFERENCES

Alvarez-Lajonchere. Personal communication. New York, 1982.
Armijo, R., Monreal, T. Estudio comparativo del aborto provocado en diversas ciudades chilenas. Revista Medica de Chile, 92, and Anales de la Sociedad Chilena de Salubridad, Santiago, Chile, 1964.
Asociacion Colombiana de Facultades de Medicina (ASCOFAME), Aborto, Dic, 1978.
Cabrera, R. Relaciones de la mortalidad infantil con la edad de la madre y numero de orden del parto; Chile, 1969-1974-1979. Revista Chilena de Obstetricia y Ginecologia 47, 1982.
CELADE, Boletin Demografico, Ano XVI, No. 32, 1983.
Departamento de Estadistica del Servicio Nacional de Salud, 1965.
Diener, W., Viel, B. El Hijo Deseado." To be published.
Gaslonde, S. Studies on Fertility and Abortion in Asuncion, Bogota, Buenos Aires, Lima, and Panama City. Scientific Publication No. 306, Epidemiology of Abortion and Practices of Fertility Regulation in Latin America, Pan American Health Organization, 1975.
Instituto Nacional de Estadisticas (INE) Chile. Informacion proporcionada a pedido in 1984. Unpublished.
Monckeberg, F., Ruimallo, J. Treatment of severe undernutrition. In B. Underwood, ed., Nutrition Policy and Intervention. MIT Press, Boston, 1982.
OPS/OMS, Conditions of Health in the Americas (1977–1980). Scientific Publication No. 427.
Ordonez, B. R., Programa del Instituto Mexicano de Seguro Social para la Prevencion del Aborto Inducido, Salud Publica No. 9, 1967.
Plaza, S., Briones, H. El aborto como problema asistencial. Revista Medica de Chile 91, 1963.
Population Reference Bureau. Cuba: The demography of revolution, 36(1), 1981.
Requena, M. A Chilean Program for Abortion Control: Fertility and Family Planning. University of Michigan Press, Ann Arbor, 1969.
Tietze, C. Induced Abortion: A World Review. Population Council, New York, 1983.
UNICEF. Dimensions of Poverty in Latin America and the Caribbean, Sanfuentes, A., and Lavados, H., Ed. Galdames, F. Santiago de Chile, 1982.

TRAINING AND DELIVERY OF ABORTION IN INDIA

Sudesh Bahl Dhall

Ticath Ram Hospital
President
Parivar Seva Sanstha
New Delhi, India

In developing countries, where the majority of the world population lives, women who already live in low socioeconomic conditions are the main victims of unregulated fertility. This lack of fertility control leads to poor health, complications in pregnancy and childbirth, general malnutrition and infection and causes an increase in maternal and perinatal mortality. Family planning has a crucial role to play in preventing unnecessary mortality.

India, with about 2 percent of the world's land area, contains about 15 percent of the world's population. 1981 Census figures show that out of 680 million, the urban population is about 22 percent. The remaining 78 percent are rural inhabitants. India is a democratic socialist country where health and family welfare are the responsibility of the government. The government is making all efforts to take health services to the people. As a concrete step to reach the goal of "Health for All" by 2000 A.D., the government of India has included primary health care, family welfare planning and nutrition in the health program of the country.

The health indices have improved considerably when compared to the early part of the present century.

Table 1: Death and Birth Rates (per 1,000 population),
India, 1920–1980

	Death Rate	Birth Rate
Pre 1920	45/1000	45/1000
1920–1960	35/1000	40/1000
1980	11.6/1000	33.2/1000

1980 Annual Growth Rate: 2.2%

The maternal mortality rate has decreased from 4.6 per 1000 live births in 1976 to less than 4 in 1980. The present position is about 3.8 per 100 live births which is very high compared to developing countries. However, as stated in the National Health Policy declaration in Parliament, India's aim is to reduce its ratio to 2—3 per 1000 live births by 2000 A.D. by recognizing and correcting the factors causing maternal deaths.

In analyzing the causes of death, we find that death after abortion is not only high but has increased from 7.9 percent in 1975 to 12.5 percent in 1980 in rural India. Many women also suffer from mental anguish and physical mutilation after abortion in a country which legalized abortion in 1972. It is estimated that five to six million abortions are performed annually in India. The number of government recognized abortion centers in 1984 was 4,553, about 20 percent located in the rural areas. The number of abortions performed in these centers in the same period was .518 million, about 10 percent of the total abortions. We assume that another 10 percent of abortions take place in private nursing homes. These are not reported. Thus, about 80 percent of abortions in India are performed by unauthorized abortionists.

The implementation of the Medical Termination of Pregnancy (MTP) Act in 1971 has created an increased awareness in the general public. Women are seeking abortions even for failure of contraceptives, a legal indication in India. Many of the general practitioners are unable to provide services when first approached and by the time a woman reaches a specialist, she is in an advanced stage of pregnancy. Fifteen to 20 percent of our women fall into this group.

Table 2: Abortion As a Cause of All Pregnancy-Related Deaths (Maternal Deaths), Rural India, 1975—1980

Year:	1975	1976	1977	1978	1979	1980
Percent of Maternal Deaths Due to Abortion	7.9	11.6	8.2	11.0	11.7	12.5

Table 3: Numbers of Medical Terminations of Pregnancies since Legalization of Abortion, India, 1972—1984

Year	No. of Institutions Approved for Elective Abortion	No. of Abortions
April '72—March '76	1,877	381,111
1976-77	2,149	178,870
1977-78	2,746	247,049
1978-79	2,765	317,732
1979-80	2,942	360,838
1980-81	3,284	388,405
1981-82	3,908	433,527
1982-83	4,170	507,984
1983-84	4,553	518,608

Table 4: Numbers and Type of Government-Recognized
Abortion Training Centers, India, 1983—84

Category	No. of Centers
Post-graduate institutes	2
Medical colleges	102
Large maternity centers/ district hospitals (postpartum centers)	57
Total:	161

Source: Government of India, Annual Report 1983-84,
p. 178.

Table 5: Number of Medical Officers Trained in
Abortion, India, 1972—1984

Period	No. Trained
1972—1982	8,498
1982-1983	970
1983-84 (1st six months)	463
Total:	9,931

Source: Government of India, Annual Report 1983-84,
p. 178.

We have found that information and access to these facilities is lacking. The number of recognized training centers for MTP in 1984 is 161. The number of medical officers trained in MTP services for the same period is 9,931. According to these figures, about 900 medical officers are trained in these 161 training centers every year or six trainees per center per year.

Out of a total of 9931 physicians, approximately 1000 are providing services in primary health centers in rural areas where 78 percent of India's population lives. In contrast nearly 9000 trained doctors are available to 22 percent of our population living in 3,300 cities and towns. This group also has access to an additional 500 private, recognized abortion institutions.

Considering the wide gap in the service delivery system, we concluded that practitioners from rural areas need to be trained in the latest safe techniques of

Table 6: Population and Abortion Services (%),
Rural and Urban India, 1984

	Rural	Urban
Distribution of Population	78%	22%
Distribution of Abortion Services	20%	80%

terminating pregnancy and in the use and dispensing of contraceptive methods to prevent further pregnancies. Practitioners should be provided with equipment and supplies to set up MTP and Family Welfare clinics in order to achieve meaningful results in the field of health and family planning.

Parivar Seva Sanstha incorporating Marie Stopes Clinics, a nongovernmental organization, of which I am the president and founding member, has taken steps to bridge the gap between the demand and supply of trained personnel in conducting abortions and providing contraceptive services.

The broad objectives of the Society are:

1. To help families protect themselves against the problems of unwanted pregnancy, maternal exhaustion, illness, and malnutrition.

2. To promote the health of children by immunization.

The Society has 13 clinics in 7 states of India and 6 more clinics will be started in the near future. Population Services, a British charity organization, assists us in many ways in the implementation of our objectives.

To solve the problem of trained medical personnel in MTP and family planning at the peripheral level, the Society started a pilot project for training from January 1983 to May 1984 with much appreciated help from the United States based Population Crisis Committee. Over 1600 applications were received. The candidates were selected on the basis of qualifications, professional experience and their locations. Preference was given to doctors of rural areas from all remote corners of India. Forty-four personnel were trained under this project. Based on the project, a 2-year pyramidal training program was initiated in January 1984. As of August 1985, 94 doctors have been trained under this project. A total of 138 doctors have been trained in the techniques of MR, MTP and contraceptive methods. The training curriculum includes:

1. A complete theoretical and practical course for correct interpretation of pelvic examination

2. Diagnosis of pregnancy and conditions like ectopic pregnancy and hydatidformole.

3. Counseling, techniques of postoperative care, legal requirements.

4. Techniques of termination of pregnancy up to 12 weeks.

5. Contraceptive methods, which is heavily stressed and, as a result, 92 percent of our clients are acceptors of some method of contraception.

6. Technical knowhow on setting up a small clinic and use and upkeep of instruments.

The training in MTP includes a complete theoretical and practical course of MR techniques with no touch technique after proper counseling so that minimum amounts of drugs are required for an outpatient procedure. Most of the MRs are performed without anesthesia. The use of general anesthesia is rare. No metal dilators are used.

After training, the physician receives a set of MR syringes and cannulae along with a syllabus. After a minimum of 25 procedures or when the doctor feels fully confident, the Society issues a certificate. Physicians return to their own localities, register themselves and start the procedure. They are asked to keep in touch in order to keep track of their progress. Two doctors trained by us, one from Ludhiana (Punjab) and another from Solan (Himachal Pradesh) have verbally reported performing 952 and about 1000 successful terminations of pregnancies respectively.

In order to expedite the process of training and to make it easier for others to go to nearby training centers, the concept of pyramidal training evolved. The doctors who are trained are expected to train other doctors in their areas in turn. An attractive incentive is paid to these pyramidal trainers. The Pyramid Project is in full swing at present and from June 1984 to August 1985, 94 doctors have been trained.

Four Pyramid Centers have been established by the trainers. From time to time we check doctors who have been trained by us to ensure adherence to the Society's medical standards. In the foreseeable future, the country will see a mushrooming of many termination of pregnancy centers and a reduction in maternal mortality and morbidity through the use of contraception and the resulting protection against further repeated and unwanted pregnancies.

On the 23d and 24th July 1985, the Society held a conference on "Innovative MTP Outreach Programs" in Delhi. The Honorable Minister of State for Health, Mr. Yogendra Makwana, in his inaugural address, said that, "Fast growing population is one of the major problems facing India. Population cannot be checked by government alone. Efforts by all, including nongovernment and voluntary organizations, are needed to accelerate the pace of the Family Planning Program".

In concluding, I wish to state that I am proud of the team which has achieved spectacular results in training other doctors in the techniques of MTP and contraceptive methods. Yet, at present, 80 percent of the population living in rural areas and urban slums only have access to backstreet abortionists. In order to have any meaningful effect on maternal mortality, morbidity, and perinatal mortality, it is necessary to provide services for this large segment of the population by expanding the MTP and contraceptive training program for private practitioners on a large scale.

LEGAL ABORTIONS IN SOCIALIST COUNTRIES OF EASTERN EUROPE:

AN EPIDEMIOLOGICAL REVIEW

K. H. Mehlan

Professor Emeritus
Rostock, German Democratic Republic

Abortion policies in the Socialist countries of Eastern Europe have undergone several major changes since 1920 when the USSR became the first country to legalize abortion on request. In 1955 the decree of 1936 outlawing abortion was repealed again and abortion was liberalized once more (abortion on request) in the USSR.

In 1956 and 1957 most socialist countries, with the exception of the German Democratic Republic (GDR) and Albania followed the example of the USSR and liberalized abortion law. In general, the liberalization of abortion laws resulted in a spectacular increase in the incidence of legal abortions during the years that followed, reflecting the replacement of unwanted birth by illegal abortions with legal abortion and the use of the new fertility freedom.

In the following tables I am using the model and the definitions initiated by Christopher Tietze.

While some countries such as the GDR reached the peak immediately, others took 12 or more years to reach their highest number of abortions. (see Figure 1)

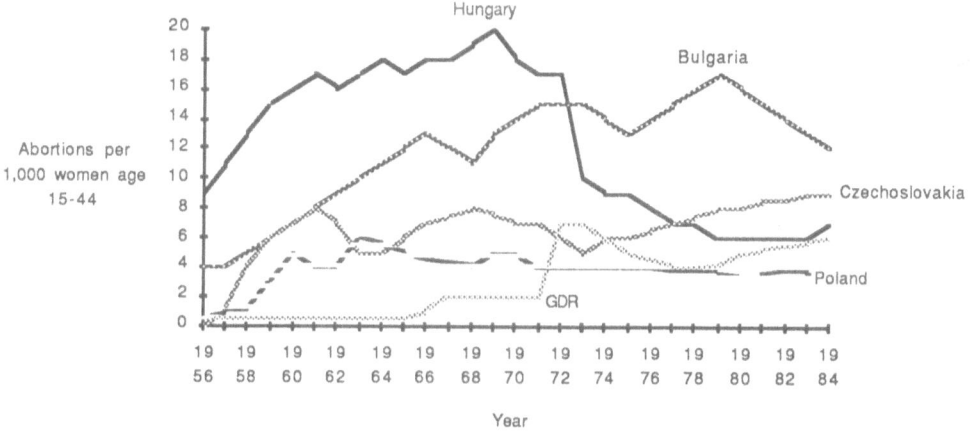

Figure 1. Abortions per 1,000 women age 15-44, in Selected Countries of Eastern Europe, 1956-1984.

BULGARIA

Abortion on request was available in Bulgaria from 1956 until 1968. The number of abortions reached nearly the number of births. The restrictive decree of 1968 had only a temporary effect followed by an upward trend in the period between 1969 and 1972 (abortion/birth ratio 1:1). The more severe restrictions in 1973 resulted in a temporary decline in the abortion rate of 10 points, but by 1982–1984 the number of abortions again reached the number of births. The restriction failed. The present stipulation is that elective abortion is available to married women with two or more living children, unmarried women without regard to age, and married women over 40 with one living child.

CZECHOSLOVAKIA

Czechoslovakia liberalized the law in 1956 to allow abortion on demand. This liberalization was followed by an eightfold rise in the number of abortions in the next year, reaching a peak after four years with 94,000 abortions in 1961 followed by a temporary decline and reaching another peak with 102,000 abortions in 1969. A new directive was issued in 1973 restricting abortion on social grounds to exceptional cases for married women without living children or with only one living child. Abortion on medical grounds is now regulated by a list of approved diagnoses. The restrictions of 1973 had less influence on the abortion figure. The abortion number increased from 81,000 to 113,000 in 1984, the abortion ratio from 280 to 510.

HUNGARY

Abortion on request was made available in 1956. Abortion figures increased rapidly and reached 207,000 in 1969. For 16 years the number of abortions exceeded the number of live births. Since January 1975, access to abortion is available only for single, divorced, separated, and widowed women, and to married women over age 40 or those who have had at least three living children. These restrictions resulted in an abrupt drop of about 40 percent, but in the last seven years, the number of abortions leveled off to around 80,000 abortions per year. By 1984, 41 percent of all known pregnancies were legally interrupted.

POLAND

Poland changed its laws in 1956 and has exemplified a stable situation over nearly 30 years. Abortion on request is permitted in in- and outpatient clinics. The abortion figure declined from 168,000 in 1956 to 133,000 in 1984 with an abortion ratio of 190 per 1,000 live births. This ratio is the lowest in all of Eastern Europe.

THE GERMAN DEMOCRATIC REPUBLIC

The German Democratic Republic extended medical indications in 1965 to take into account the woman's social environment. In 1972, abortion on request during the first trimester of pregnancy was authorized to be available for all women free of charge in a gynecological hospital. Abortions must be performed within one week after application. In 1972 there was a fivefold increase in the number of abortions. (see Figure 2)

Influenced by social and political measures and the sharp increase in the use of effective contraceptives, the abortion ratio per 1,000 live births dropped from 620 in 1972 to 360 in 1980. In the last four years the abortion ratio increased slowly up to 411 in 1984 along with an increasing number of live births and an increase in fertility rate.

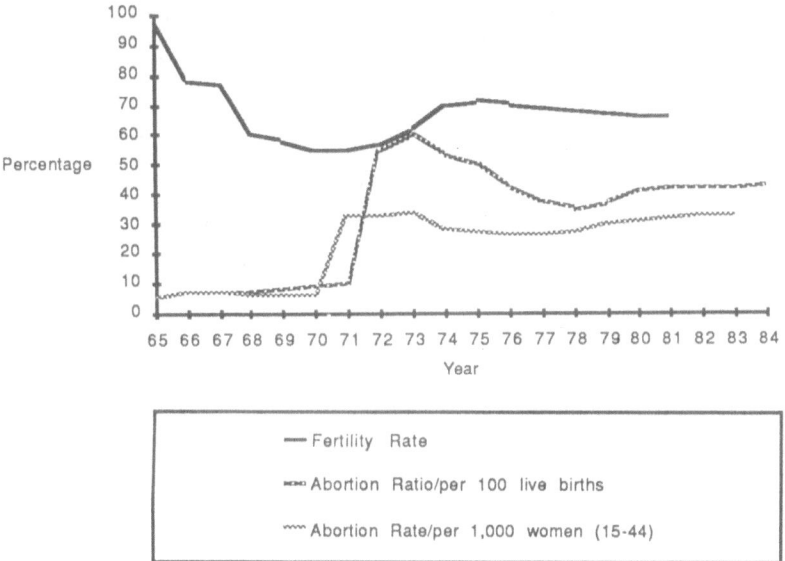

Figure 2. Abortion Rate and Ratio and Fertility Role, District of Rostock, German Democratic Republic, 1965-84.

Table 1: Legal Abortions per 1,000 Women Age 15—44,
Selected Socialist Countries, 1956—1984

Year	Bulgaria	CSSR	GDR	Hungary	Poland
1956	14	12	3	464	16
1960	400	405	3	1,129	337
1964	719	298	7	1,393	312
1968	641	456	83	1,310	289
1972	986	347	590	1,161	230
1976	880	305	418	505	215
1980	914	413	361	620	199
1984	950	510	411	691	190

Table 2: Legal Abortions, German Democratic Republic, 1972—1984

Year	Total (in 1,000s)	% of Base Year (1972)	Rate (per 1,000 women 15—44)	Ratio (per 100 live births)
1972	114.0	= 100	33	57
1973	110.8		32	62
1974	99.7		29	56
1975	87.8		25	48
1976	81.9		23	42
1977	78.0	= 68	22	35
1978	76.2	= 66	22	33
1980	80.6		24	36
1982	90.4		25	38
1984	96.2	= 84	26	41

Table 3: Legal Abortions, Selected Socialist Countries, 1967, 1976, and 1984

Countries	Year	Total (in 1,000s)	Rate (per 1,000 women 15–44)	Ratio (per 100 live births)
Bulgaria	1967	98.2	52	79
	1976	123.4	65	86
	1984	113.0	62	95
Czechoslovakia	1967	96.4	45	31
	1976	84.6	27	30
	1984	113.2	34	51
German Democratic Republic	1967	20.0	5	8
	1976	81.9	23	42
	1984	96.2	26	41
Hungary	1967	187.5	83	126
	1976	94.7	42	51
	1984	82.2	37	61
Poland	1967	146.1	20	28
	1975	138.6	18	22
	1984	133.0	16	19

USSR

Abortion on request was reinstituted in the USSR in 1955 for all women during the first trimester. Exact figures for the Soviet Union as a whole are not available. There are investigations of scientists in different years and regions. The estimates range from 6.5 million (Dr. Bloshansky) to 10 million legal abortions in 1970 (IPPF statement) to 16.5 million in 1980 (Davis and Serenko). Sadvokassova dealt with the epidemiology of abortion for more than 20 years and came to the result that in the bigger cities there are on an average 2 or 3 abortions for each birth, while the ratio is one to one in the rural areas. These figures correspond to an abortion ratio of 1,600 per 1,000 live births.

MEDICAL EXPERIENCE WITH ABORTION AFTER

LEGALIZATION IN WESTERN EUROPE

Evert Ketting

Director of Research
STIMEZO Netherland
(National Abortion Federation of the Netherlands)
Zeist, The Netherlands

INTRODUCTION

Until now there has been no attempt in Western Europe to undertake a comprehensive international comparative study on the medical aspects of abortion care. One of the rare exceptions to the general lack of exchange of epidemiological data and clinical experience has been a conference on second-trimester abortions which was organized at the University of Leiden, Holland, in 1980 (Keirse et al., 1982). In addition, the late Christopher Tietze has included European epidemiological data on some medical aspects in his worldwide surveys on abortion (Tietze, 1983). This general lack of exchange of relevant medical information and experience is a serious problem which hampers the development and general acceptance of simple, inexpensive, convenient, and safe abortion procedures. One example can be found in southern Germany, where the local governments are still withholding outpatient services with the argument that those procedures would not be safe (Bericht, 1980; Ketting and van Praag, 1985). It is therefore absolutely necessary that initiatives be taken to organize the exchange of information systematically, preferably by means of an international journal.

THE ATTITUDES OF THE MEDICAL PROFESSION

In the evaluation of medical experience with abortion in Western Europe the attitude of the medical profession should be a major concern. We always tend to look at what doctors are doing in this field, but it may be more useful to focus on what they are not doing. A major problem is that many doctors are reluctant or refuse to perform abortions and sometimes this is quite understandable. In Italy, for instance, almost three-quarters of all doctors are officially registered as conscientious objectors to abortion (Delpierre, 1979). In West Germany 62 percent of the heads of gynecological departments do not accept all legal indications for abortion (Bericht, 1980), a remarkable figure in view of the fact that West Germany already has the most restrictive of all new abortion laws in Western Europe (Ketting and van Praag, 1985).

In France so many doctors in hospitals were unwilling to perform abortions that in 1982 the government decided to compel public hospitals to appoint doctors who were willing and able to perform abortions (Ministere de la Sante, 1982). In Austria abortion has such a negative image and connotes such taboo that a doctor who is known as an abortionist has little chance to have a professional career

(Ketting and van Praag, 1985). The same is true in many parts of West Germany. Until now it has been almost impossible to find German doctors who are prepared to work in an independent clinic, such as those of Pro Familia, where they will be publicly known to perform abortions. Some doctors want to perform abortions as long as they are not publicly known to do so. As a consequence, several Dutch doctors have been hired to work there. Thus, one of the main medical problems with abortion in Western Europe is to find doctors who are willing to perform them.

EPIDEMIOLOGY OF ABORTION IN WESTERN EUROPE

Examining the major epidemiological data on abortion in Western Europe, there can be no doubt that legalization of abortion is associated with a sharp decrease in the number of complications. This is best exemplified by rates of fatal complications as other complications are difficult to compare.

The downward trend in complications can probably be explained by a combination of three factors. First, legalization has, by increasing the accessibility of abortion services, resulted in a tremendous reduction in the mean gestational age at abor-

Table 1. Abortion Mortality per 100,000 in Selected Western
European Countries and the U.S.A., 1953—1980

Country	Years	No. of Deaths	Mortality Rate per 100,000 Abortions
Denmark	1953—57	16	68
	1961—66	9	33
	1967—80	4	1.6
Sweden	1949—53	27	96
	1954—63	21	60
	1964—79	8	2.4
England and Wales	1968—69	20	26
	1970—72	43	12
	1973—78	31	3.5
	1979—80	5	1.6
W. Germany	1976—77	10	14.9
	1978—80	1	0.8
	1980—83	8	3.0
Netherlands	1970—74	2	0.8
	1975—79	0	0
	1980—84	1	0.4
France	1970	50	--
	1974	26	--
	1977	9	--
U.S.A.	1963—68	7	72
	1970—73	139	6.9
	1974—77	82	1.9
	1978—80	33	0.7

Sources: Tietze, 1981, 1983; Ketting and van Praag, 1985; Statistisches Bundesamt 1977—1984.

tion. Sweden has been the most striking example in this respect, but it has occurred in other countries as well.

The percentage of late abortions has leveled off at a comparatively high level in England and West Germany, most likely caused by the rather complicated procedures required of women before actually obtaining an abortion (Ketting and van Praag, 1985).

It is well known that the risk of complications rises sharply with increasing pregnancy duration, as is illustrated by Table 3.

The second factor that has contributed to the decrease in complication rates is the use of modern, safer methods. It is by now almost universally accepted that suction or vacuum aspiration is the safest method of abortion in the first trimester of pregnancy. This is confirmed by recent German data that show a national complication rate of 3.8 per 100 curettage abortions compared to a rate of 1.6 for vacuum aspiration (Statistisches Bundesamt, 1984).

Despite these findings some countries, notably Italy, West Germany, and Denmark, continue to have an unacceptably high proportion of first-trimester abortions performed by means of sharp curettage, as shown in Table 4.

The growing knowledge and experience of doctors and auxiliary personnel are a third reason for the decrease in complication rates.

It is difficult to illustrate this growing experience by means of adequate data, but it is interesting to note that complication rates in the more specialized free-

Table 2: Percentage of Abortions Performed at More than 12 Weeks (from LMP) Gestation in Selected Western European Countries and the U.S.A.

Country	Year	% at More Than 12 Weeks Gestation
Sweden	1968	57.1
	1975	7.0
	1982	4.7
England and Wales	1968	38.0
	1975	17.4
	1982	14.3
West Germany	1976	44.5
(12 weeks or more)	1980	25.9
	1983	19.1
	1984	19.2
Finland	1975	13.2
	1978	9.5
	1980	4.5
U.S.A.	1973	14.5
	1977	8.9
	1980	8.7

Sources: Tietze, 1983; OPCS, 1983 (England and Wales); Stat. Bundesamt 1977–1985 (W. Germany).

Table 3: Complication Rate per 100 Abortions by
Pregnancy Duration in the U.S.A. and Denmark

Weeks of Pregnancy Duration	Complication Rate U.S.A. 1971–1975/Denmark 1980	
	Major Complications	All Complications
6 or fewer	.44	3.3
7–8	.29	3.3
9–10	.34	3.4
11–12	.41	5.0
13–14	.69	6.5
15–16	1.44	9.4
17–20	1.96	12.6
21 or more	1.71	--

Sources: Tietze, 1983; Sundhedsstyrelsen, 1984.

Table 4: Abortion during the First Trimester of Pregnancy
by Method in Five Countries

Country	Method			
	Vacuum Asp.	Curet- tage	Med. Induction	Other Methods
Sweden 1980	98.6	.5	.5	.5
Denmark 1980	89.9	9.5	.2	.2
Denmark 1983	92.6	7.1	.1	.2
England & Wales 1980	93.2	5.0	1.5	.3
West Germany 1980*	76.1	22.1	1.2	.6
West Germany 1983*	79.7	18.4	1.6	.2
U.S.A. 1976	95.0	4.4	.4	.1
Italy 1983**	74.9	24.5	.6	

Sources: Socialstyrelsen, 1982 (Sweden); Sundhedsstyrelsen, 1982 (Denmark); OPCS, 1982 (England); Stat. Bundesamt 1981, 1984 (W. Germany); CDC, 1978 (U.S.A.); Spinelli et al., 1985 (Italy).
* Abortions 11 weeks since LMP.
** All abortions, including 0.9% over 12 weeks.

standing clinics are generally lower than in general hospitals. In the U.S. it has been shown that this difference disappears after controlling the data for preexisting complications (Grimes, 1981).

A lower fatal complication risk in clinics might also be due to the fact that the average annual number of abortions performed by doctors in general hospitals is much lower than that for clinics. For instance, in England the fatal complication rate in hospitals has been eight times higher in hospitals than in clinics during the past decade. In Holland, two of the three deaths that have occurred there since 1970 took place in hospitals, although only about 10 percent of all abortions are performed there. In both cases the women were not referred to the hospital because of preexisting complications.

From a medical point of view it must be regretted that several European governments, i.e., France, Italy, Denmark, and large parts of West Germany, have legally prevented the establishment of specialized abortion facilities (Ketting and van Praag, 1985). In the Netherlands, England, and the U.S.A most abortions are now performed in well-equipped and specialized clinics, while in West Germany about half of the operations take place in hospitals and the other half in private doctors' offices (Statistisches Bundesamt, 1984). The specialized clinic, which appears to be the most suitable set-up, is very difficult to organize because of legal, administrative, and attitudinal barriers.

SUMMARY

From a medical point of view the development of abortion services has been generally positive in Western Europe. However, some further changes are still needed:

1. There should be more systematic exchange of information and experience.

2. In some countries, notably England and West Germany, the accessibility of abortion services should be increased and complicated administrative barriers need to be removed in order to decrease the number of late abortions.

3. In some countries, and again notably West Germany, the use of modern and safe methods should be encouraged.

4. Legal or administrative barriers that hamper the development of specialized outpatient services should be removed.

REFERENCES

Bericht der "Kommission zur Auswertung der Erfahrungen mit dem reformierten Par. 218 des Strafgesetzbuches." Unterrichtung durch die Bundesregierung, Deutscher Bundestag, Drucksache 8/3630 vom 31 Januar 1980.
Centers for Disease Control (CDC). Abortion surveillance 1976. DHHS, Atlanta, 1978.
Delpierre, G. In G. Halimi, Choisir de donner la vie. Colloque Internationale de "Choisir" des 5, 6, 7 october 1979 a l'Unesco. Gallimard, Paris, 1979.
Grimes, D. A., Cates, W., and Selik, R. Abortion facilities and risk of death. Family Planning Perspectives 13(1):30, 1981.
Keirse, M. J. C. N., Bennebroek Gravenhorst, J., van Lith, D. A. F., et al., eds. Second Trimester Pregnancy Termination. Leiden University Press, The Hague, 1982.
Ketting, E., van Praag, P. Schwangerschaftsabbruch, Gesetz und Praxis im internationalen Vergleich. DGVT-Verlag, Tubingen, 1985.
Ministere de la Sante. Circulaire no. 12-82 du 12 octobre relative a l'amelioration de l'information et de la prescription de la contraception et de la pratique des interruptions volontaires de grossesse dans les etablissements publics, Paris. 1982.
Office of Population Censuses and Surveys (OPCS). Monitor: Legal abortions 1982. HMSO, London, 1983.
Spinelli, A., Pediconi, M., Grandolfo, M. E., et al. Legal Abortion in Italy--1983. Instituto Superiore di Sanita, Rome, 1985.
Statistisches Bundesamt. Schwangerschaftsabbrueche 1976–1984 (several volumes). Wiesbaden, 1977–1985.
Sundhedsstyrelsen. Statistik om praevention og aborter, 1981. Copenhagen, 1982.

Sundhedsstyrelsen. Statistik om praevention og aborter, 1983 (1982). Copenhagen, 1984.

Tietze, C. Induced Abortion: A World Review, 1981. The Population Council, New York, 1981.

Tietze, C. Induced Abortion: A World Review, 1983. The Population Council, New York, 1983.

THE EFFECTS OF LEGISLATION OF ABORTION

ON MATERNAL AND PERINATAL OUTCOME

Kuldip Singh
Lecturer

Osborn Viegas,
Senior Lecturer

S. S. Ratnam
Professor and Head

Department of Obstetrics and Gynecology
National University Hospital
National University of Singapore
Singapore, Republic of Singapore

ABSTRACT

In general, national family planning programs in several countries have relied largely on voluntary acceptance of contraception as a means of regulating population growth. However, it is well known that voluntary family planning programs, even when highly successful, may often fail to achieve demographic goals such as zero growth. In these situations, measures have been recommended that 'go beyond family planning' in an attempt to influence the number of children couples choose to have. Singapore has successfully used legislation to achieve its desired demographic changes. This success, within a legal framework, is unique and may be used as a model for other countries where voluntary participation in national family planning programs has failed.

Abortion-related maternal mortality may be compared appropriately with the risk to life associated with carrying a pregnancy to term. In Singapore, the overall mortality following abortion has declined substantially--from 15 abortion related deaths between 1968–1970 to no abortion related deaths in the years 1980–1983. We believe this decline is due to the replacement of illegal by legal abortions (enhanced by liberalized legislation) and improvements in the quality of services and efficient treatment of complications.

Furthermore, with an increase in the number of legal abortions, the crude birth rate has shown a dramatic decline from 29.5 per 1,000 population in 1965 to 16.2 per 1,000 in 1983. This has resulted in smaller family sizes with greater access to socio-economic assets of the country leading to healthier mothers and a significant improvement in their reproductive performance. The perinatal mortality has declined from 25.5 per 1,000 in 1965 to 10.6 per 1,000 in 1983. Similarly the infant mortality rate has declined from 26.3 in 1965 to 9.4 per 1,000 in 1983.

INTRODUCTION

In general, national family planning programs in several countries, even those with explicit demographic goals, have relied largely on voluntary acceptance of contraception. However, it is well known that voluntary family planning programs, even when highly successful, may often fail to achieve demographic goals such as zero growth (David and Kingsley, 1967). In these situations, measures have been recommended that 'go beyond family planning' in an attempt to influence the number of children couples choose to have (Berdson, 1969a). Singapore is an example of a country that has gone well beyond family planning to reach its population objectives. Since 1966, the Singapore national family planning and population program has had very clear demographic goals i.e., to reach replacement reproduction by 1980 and achieve zero population growth by 2030 (Kee and Loh, 1973). To promote these goals the Government of Singapore has used legislation to discourage births above given birth orders: Initially fourth births and later third births. To enhance the impact of these laws on population control, the Government of Singapore has introduced a series of incentives and disincentives--indeed Singapore is the first nation to have implemented primarily disincentives in the family reduction programs. A list of these incentives and disincentives is given in Table 1. Although these disincentives are tangible negative sanctions, it must be stressed that the Government does not impose legal punitive measures on those not restricting family size to the stipulated two.

Table 1: Disincentive and Incentive Policies to Reduce Fertility

Disincentives	Incentives
1. Increasing accouchement charges for increasing birth orders.	1. Waivers of delivery charges.
2. Low school admission priority for families with 3 or more children.	2. Paid medical leave for mothers undergoing sterilization after delivery of third or subsequent children.
3. No paid maternity leave for delivery of third and subsequent children.	3. Monetary stipends in some cases where sexual sterilization is undertaken by the mother after the first or second child.
4. Tax relief for the first 3 children only.	4. Continuation of employment for non-Singaporeans. Only if both partners undergo sexual sterilization after delivery of the second child.
5. Low housing subsidy allocation priority for families with 3 or more children.	

Table 2: Legalized Abortion Statistics for Singapore

Year	1970	71	72	73	74	75	76	77	78	79	80	81	82	83
Number of abortions	1,913	3,407	3,806	5,252	7,175	12,703	15,496	16,443	17,246	16,999	18,219	18,890	19,910	19,000
Rates per 1,000 women aged 15-44 yrs.	4.2	7.2	7.7	10.3	13.6	23.3	27.5	28.3	28.4	27.1	28.4	28.8	28.6	28.6
Legal abortion/ livebirths (%)	4.1	7.2	7.7	10.9	16.6	32.2	36.2	42.9	43.7	41.7	44.2	44.7	44.8	46.8

In addition abortion laws have been liberalized to a point where termination of pregnancy is now "available on demand" up to the 24th week of pregnancy. This liberalization has resulted in improvements in obstetric outcome for mother and child and furthermore has enabled smaller family units to enjoy a much more acceptable standard of living.

The progressive liberalization of abortion laws since 1966 is outlined below.

ABORTION

Before 1967: Legal abortion restricted to those cases where maternal life was endangered.

1967: Medical Committee of the National Family Planning and Population Board set up. Extended abortion to (1) those eugenic cases e.g., with congenital fetal malformations and (2) those cases where the mother was a victim of sex crime or of intercourse with a mentally insane or feeble minded person.

1968: First Abortion Bill. Abortion further liberalized to include those cases deemed unsuitable for continuing pregnancy for family, social and economic reasons. This facility was only available for those women who were residents of Singapore for more than four months prior to the abortion.

1974: New Abortion Act. This law made it possible for abortions to be performed up to 24 weeks of pregnancy by a registered medical practitioner with prescribed qualifications and/or experience in a government hospital or in an approved institution at the written request of the woman.

ABORTION RATES IN SINGAPORE

The legalization of abortions in Singapore has had a dramatic effect on population structure. During the period 1970 to 1983, 176,459 legal abortions have been documented. The proportion of legal abortions to live births has also increased progressively from 4.1 percent in 1970 to 46.8 percent in 1983 (Table 2).

LEGALIZED ABORTION: IMPACT ON MATERNAL MORTALITY

Family planning meets individual and community needs. Although some couples in developing countries want large families, many men and women want to control their fertility. In particular, many have personal reasons for wanting to prevent the very pregnancies that coincidentally pose the greatest health risks. Evidence of the desire to prevent births is seen in survey results and in levels of illegal abortion (CAPMAS, 1983). Figure 1 shows reported deaths from illegal abortion in various countries. These numbers do not necessarily show which countries have the highest rates (they may just have a more accurate reporting system) and all of these rates are probably underestimates. However it does give some picture of illegal abortion as a public health problem.

In countries, where abortion is legal, for example Canada, the United States, Japan and several other nations--deaths from illegal abortions are almost unknown now--less than one death per million women aged 15—44 years (Tietze, 1981).

The potential for preventing deaths from illegal abortion through family planning is clearly very great since these pregnancies are unwanted. This has been demonstrated in a number of countries including the United States, United Kingdom and Chile (Liskin, 1980; Cales et al., 1978; WHO, 1978). For example, in Chile, where abortions are still illegal, contraceptive use increased from 3.2 percent to 23 percent between 1964 and 1978. At the same time the number of

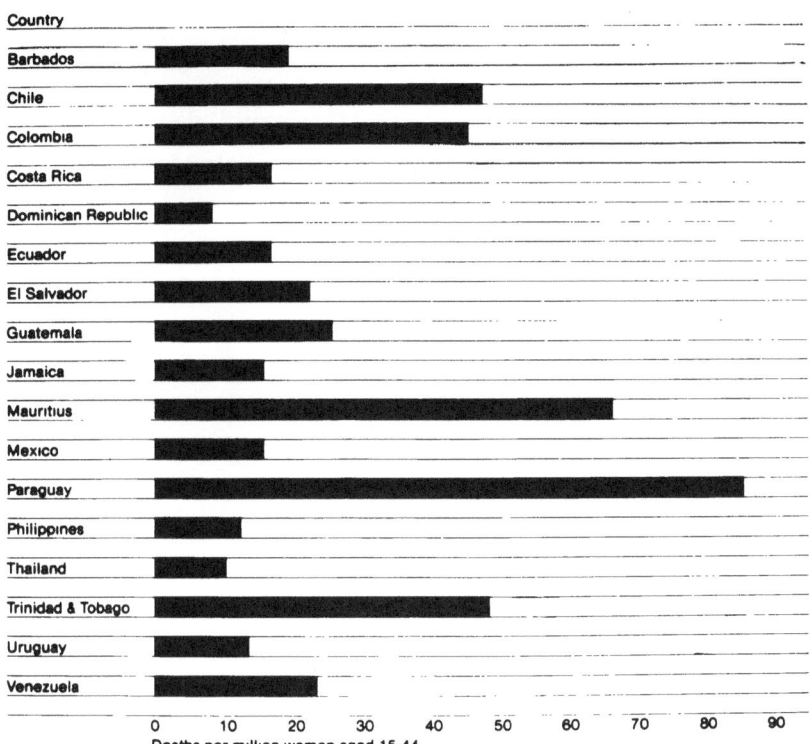

Country
Barbados
Chile
Colombia
Costa Rica
Dominican Republic
Ecuador
El Salvador
Guatemala
Jamaica
Mauritius
Mexico
Paraguay
Philippines
Thailand
Trinidad & Tobago
Uruguay
Venezuela

0   10   20   30   40   50   60   70   80   90
Deaths per million women aged 15-44

Fig. 1:   Annual Deaths from Illegal Abortion, in Various
Countries, 1970.
Source: Family Planning--its impact on the health of
women and children, Center for Population and Family
Health, Faculty of Medicine, Columbia University, New
York, 1983.

hospitalization due to complications from abortion fell by one third (Figure 2).
Furthermore, as shown in Figure 3, the rate of maternal mortality due to abortions
declined from 118 per 100,000 live births to 20 per 100,000 live births (Lincoln,
1984). This decline not only saved many women from suffering and death, but it
has also allowed such valuable hospital resources as blood supplies, antibiotics, bed
space and staff time to be used to care for other people in need. This is important
in developing countries where medical resources are scarce.

Similarly, in Singapore the liberalization of abortion legislation in 1970 and
the availability of abortion on demand for pregnancies up to 24 weeks in 1974 has
shown a progressive fall in the abortion deaths from 15 in 1968–1970 to 9 in
1974–1976, a decline of 40 percent (Lim, et al., 1979). This is substantiated by the
increase in the number of legalized abortion over the period 1971–1979. A more
recent analysis of data shows that there were no abortion related deaths in the
years 1979–83 (Figure 4).

DECLINE IN BIRTH RATES

The crude birth rate in Singapore was 42.7 per 1,000 population in 1957. It
has declined sharply since then. At the end of 1965 the crude birth rate was around

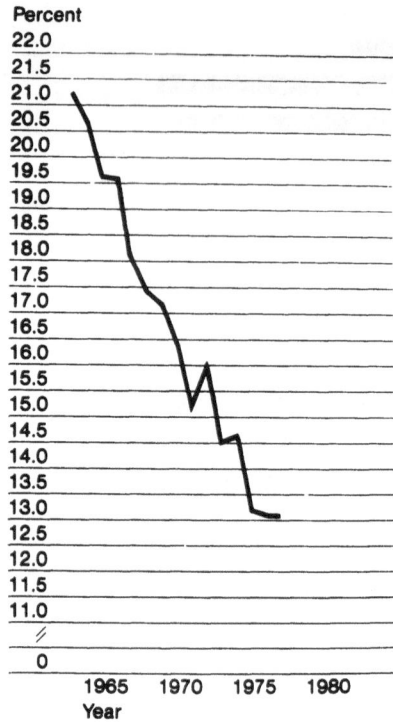

Percent

1965   1970   1975   1980
Year

Fig. 2:   Percent of all Obstetric Hospitalizations that were
due to Abortion, Chile, 1964–1968.
Source: Family Planning--its impact on the health of
women and children, Center for Population and Family
Health, Faculty of Medicine, Columbia University, New
York, 1983.

29.5 per 1,000 population but, with the introduction of the National family planning
program in 1966, the rate fell to around 20 per 1,000 in 1970. It was at this stage
that abortion was legalized and thereafter the crude birth rate fell rapidly so that
in 1983 it was 16.2 per 1,000 population (Figure 5) (Singapore, 1968–1984).

IMPROVEMENT IN PERINATAL AND INFANT MORTALITY RATES

The change in childbearing resulting from the introduction of family planning
has shown a dramatic reduction of both infant and maternal mortality all over the
world.

In Singapore perinatal mortality was 28.3 per 1,000 total live births and stillbirths in 1957. It showed a fall to 25.5 per 1,000 in 1965. With the introduction of
the National Family Planning Program in 1966 and liberalization of abortion in
1974 it has decreased sharply to 10.6 in 1983 (Figure 5). This trend is also shown in
the infant mortality rates. The infant mortality rate was 41.4 per 1,000 live births
in 1957 and 26.3 in 1965. With the introduction of family planning and legalized
abortion it has been more significantly reduced so that in 1983, the infant mortality rate for Singapore was 9.4 per 1,000 live births (Singapore, 1968; Singapore,
1982).

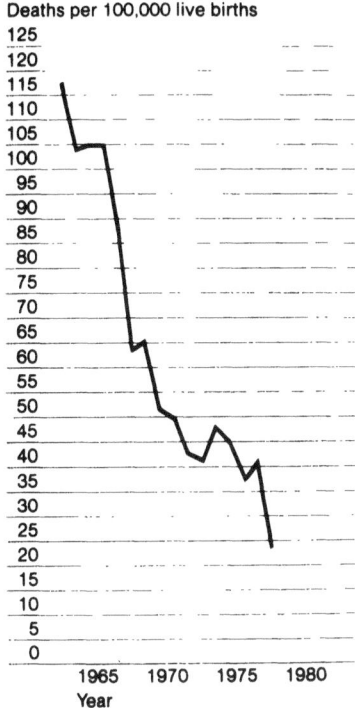

Deaths per 100,000 live births

Fig. 3: Maternal Deaths due to Abortion in Chile, 1964–
1979.
Source: Family Planning--its impact on the health of
women and children, Center for Population and Family
Health, Faculty of Medicine, Columbia University, New
York, 1983.

The success of the national family planning program and the legislation of
abortion in Singapore have been largely responsible for the decline in maternal,
perinatal and infant deaths, but the role of the overall improvement of the maternal educational status and the socio-economic circumstances of the family cannot
be overlooked. The per capita gross national product in Singapore has increased
from 3,849 Singapore dollars in 1973 to 11,031 Singapore dollars in 1983.

TOTAL FERTILITY RATES

The fertility rate provides an indicator of the number of children a woman
will have during her entire reproductive life span on the basis of the existing
fertility rate at the time of the study.

In Singapore the decrease in fertility trends was noted from 1957. During the
period 1957–1965 the total fertility rate declined from 6.4 to 4.6 per woman. With
the introduction of the national family planning program in 1966, the decline in
fertility accelerated especially during the period 1966–1970 so that in 1970, the
total fertility rate was 3.1 per woman. This general declining trend in fertility has
continued and in 1983, was 1.6 (Figure 6) (Singapore, 1968; 1982; Bangladesh, 1978;
Population Ref. Bureau, 1981).

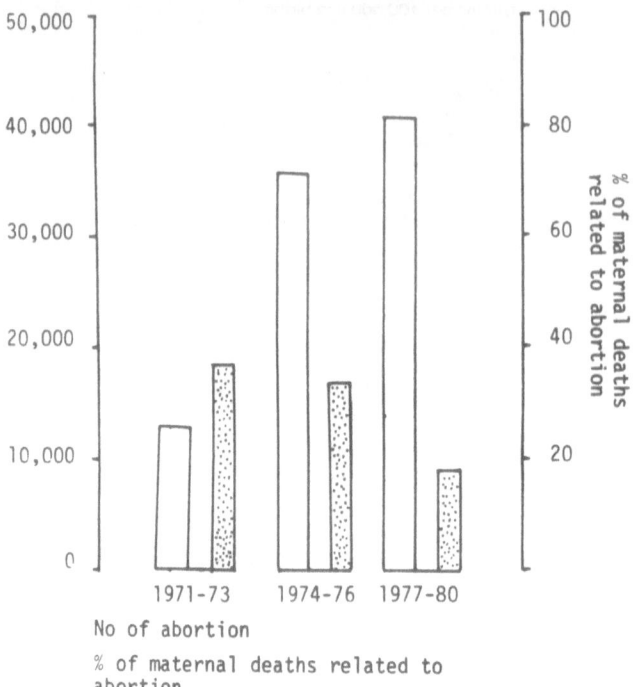

Fig. 4:   Trends in Legalized Abortion in Singapore and Abortion related Maternal Deaths, 1971-1980.
Source: Lim et al., 1979.

An even more important demographic change occurred among the more afflu-
ent and educated Singaporean. Whereas the original intention was to reduce the
net reproductive rate to one, the rate fell to 0.8 in 1980 with mainly the higher
socioeconomic class causing this drop. As a result of this change, the government
brought about a selective priority scheme to encourage graduate females to have
three children instead of two. From January 1984, these mothers were promised
first priority in the registration for the school of their choice and more favorable
income tax relief benefits. However, this selective policy created social dissatis-
faction and is to be discontinued in March 1986. This reversal serves to emphasize
the need for such policies to be applied across the board and with fairness if
equitable compliance is to be achieved.

CONCLUSION

The successful legalization of abortion in Singapore has clearly helped the
government to achieve the desired demographic changes within this densely popu-
lated city state. The restriction of population has allowed for substantial improvement in the socioeconomic standard of every Singaporean reflected by the escalating per capita Gross National Product seen during the last decade.

Induced abortion as a measure for population control is now generally accepted in Singapore and with the advances in available techniques, it has become a
much less hazardous procedure.

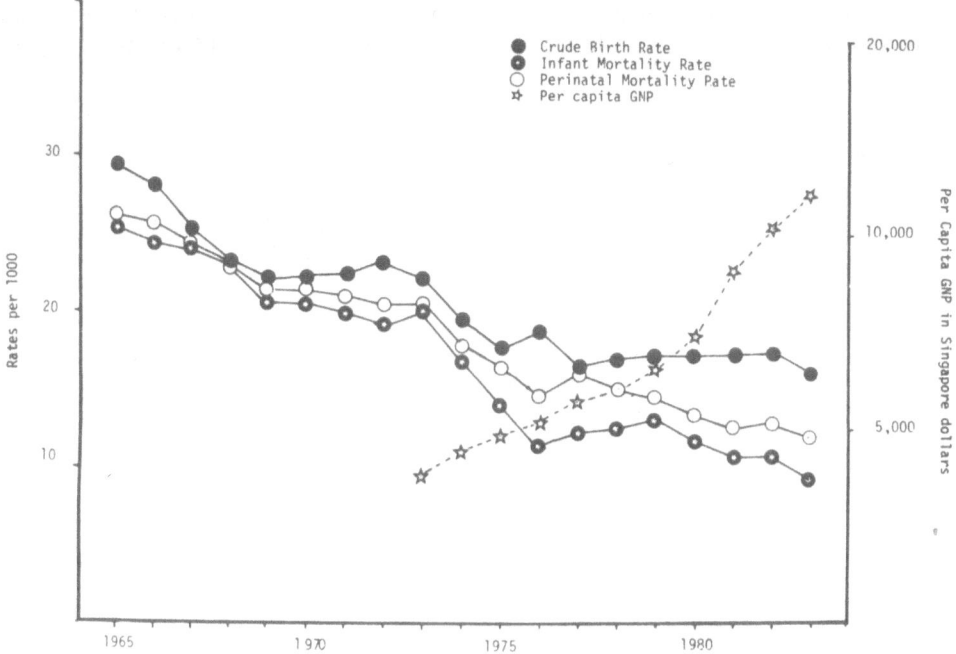

Fig. 5: Crude Birth Rates, Infant Mortality Rate and perinatal Mortality Rates for Singapore, 1965—1983, with change
in per capita GNP, 1973—1983.
Source: Singapore Family Planning and Population Board
Annual Reports, 1984.

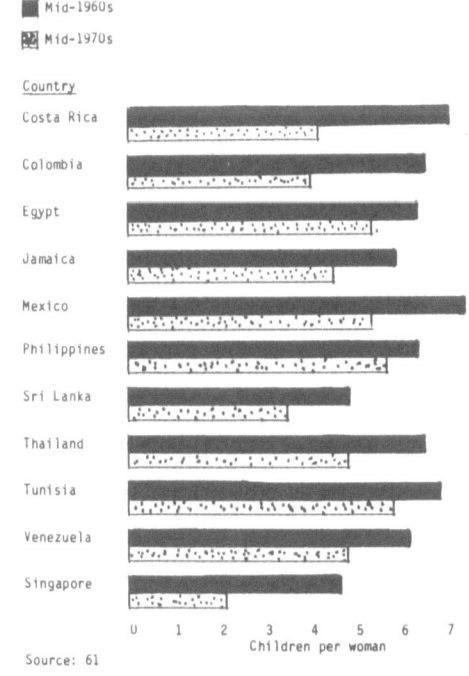

Fig. 6: Total Fertility Rates in Mid 1960, Mid 1970, in 11
Countries.
Source: Population Reference Bureau, 1983.

Liberal abortion laws have also abolished criminal abortion with its attendant risks to mothers and made low-cost abortion readily available to all Singapore women.

Singapore's success in achieving its demographic goals within a legal framework is unique and can be used as a model for other countries where voluntary participation in national family planning programs has failed. Unfortunately, however, this may not apply to some developing countries where size, rural conditions, low levels of literacy and sparse economic reserves may prove to be major setbacks in the implementation of such population policies.

REFERENCES

Bangladesh Fertility Survey 1975—1976. Ministry of Health and Population Control. Population Control and Family Planning Division, Government of the People's Republic of Bangladesh, First Report, Dhaka, 1978.

Berelson, B. Beyond family planning. Studies in Family Planning 38:1, 1969.

Cates, W., Rochat, R. W., Grimes, D. A., et al. Legalized abortion: Effect on national trends of maternal and abortion-related mortality (1940 through 1976). American Journal of Obstetrics and Gynecology 132(2):211, 1978.

David and Kingsley. Population policy: Will the current programs succeed? Science 58:730, 1967.

Egypt. Central Agency for Public Mobilization and Statistics (CAPMAS). The Egyptian Fertility Survey 1980, volume 4. Cairo, World Fertility Survey p. 357, 1983.

Kee, W. F., Loh, M. In: Family planning programs. World Review eds. W. B. Watson and R. J. Laphan. Studies in Family Planning 6;8:136, 1973.

Lim, L. S., Cheng, M. C. E., Rauff, M., Ratnam, S. S. Abortion deaths in Singapore 1968—1967, Singapore Medical Journal 20:391, 1979.

Lincoln, R. FDA committee: no support for pill-breast cancer link, but cervical cancer connection more ambiguous. International Family Planning Perspectives 10:27, 1984.

Liskin, L. S. Complications of abortions in developing countries. Population Reports, Series F, 6:105, July 1980.

Population Reference Bureau, World Fertility: A chart of age--specific fertility rates for 120 countries. Washington D.C., January 1981.

Singapore Family Planning and Population Board Annual Reports, 1968—1984.

Statistics from Registrar of Births and Deaths, Singapore, 1982—1983.

Tietze, C. Induced Abortion: A World Review. The Population Council, New York, 1981.

World Health Organization (WHO), Induced abortion: Report of a WHO scientific group, WHO Technical Report Series No. 623, Geneva, 1978.

MEDICAL PRACTICE AFTER LEGALIZATION OF ABORTION:

THE CHINESE EXPERIENCE

Yan Ren-Ying
Beijing Medical University
Beijing, People's Republic of China

ABSTRACT

Induced abortion has been legalized since the early 1950s in the People's Republic of China. The procedure is freely available to women at all administrative levels of hospitals and clinics in both urban and rural areas. Most abortions have been performed on an outpatient basis by trained paramedics, such as nurses, midwives, and barefoot doctors, with supervision by medical doctors. Suction and curettage, dilatation and evacuation, and intra-amniotic instillation are the main methods of abortion currently used. Patients with complications associated with the procedure are treated or hospitalized free of charge. In 1982, a sample survey of childbearing married women aged below 50 conducted in Beijing City shows that the annual rate of abortion was 67 per 1,000 respondents, and the abortion ratio was 83 per 100 live births in 1982; 11.7 percent of respondents' last abortions were performed after 12 weeks of gestation; and 1.4 percent of respondents were hospitalized after their last abortion because of having had serious symptoms, such as bleeding, infection, and abdominal pain, associated with the abortions. The prevalence and incidence, weeks of gestation, and short-term complications associated with induced abortion obtained from the Beijing survey are further classified by sociodemographic characteristics of respondents, and are also compared with those of other countries where the data are available.

INTRODUCTION

In old China, women were discriminated in many respects; they were mostly illiterate, socially subject to and economically dependent on men. With the founding of the People's Republic of China, for the first time women were given equal rights. More and more women accepted education, began to walk out of their homes, and took up various posts. Still, many obstacles prevent women from raising their status. Among others, unplanned pregnancy has been a serious hindrance to their progress. In order to reduce the number of unplanned pregnancies, and give women the right to terminate unwanted pregnancies, the government began in the early 1950s to advocate contraceptive practice by making contraceptive supply and services available to married couples. In 1953, the government passed a law legalizing induced abortion when requested by the couple.

Since legalization of abortion, the procedure has been widely and freely available to women in hospitals and clinics in the People's Republic of China. In urban areas, abortion is performed in city, district, and regional hospitals, while in rural villages women can obtain the abortion in county and township (commune) hospitals, and possibly at the local barefoot doctor's clinic if the expertise is available. In both urban and rural areas, most abortions are performed on an outpatient basis by trained paramedics such as a nurse, midwife, and barefoot doctor, with supervision by medical doctors.

Early abortions are usually performed by paramedics who have received special training and have been scrutinized for their technical proficiency before they are allowed to do the operation independently. However, for the sake of safety, all mid-trimester abortions are performed only in hospital by medical doctors. Since safety is considered the first priority, strict observance of operating protocol is demanded in the process of the procedure to enforce quality control, and major complications have to be discussed by experts so that adequate measures can be taken to protect the health of the patients.

In order to safeguard post-operative recovery, the government suggests that post-operative sick leave of two weeks be given to all women after an abortion, and an additional two days be given to those who have an IUD inserted right after the abortion. Those who have post-abortal sterilization are entitled to a month of sick leave. Not only is abortion performed free of charge for every woman, those with complications are treated or hospitalized at no cost to the individual.

The technique used for abortion depends on the period of gestation. Vacuum aspiration and curettage is used for pregnancies under 11 weeks. Suction machines are made especially for this purpose. If machines are not available, negative pressure produced in a half-liter rubber-stop bottle can serve the same purpose. Usually anesthesia is not necessary, and the typical amount of bleeding is about 20 ml. Dilatation and evacuation is the usual procedure for terminating pregnancies between 11 and 14 weeks. Preliminary insertion of a rubber catheter to soften the cervix has proven to be very effective to prevent cervical laceration. When gestation has gone beyond 14 weeks, it is preferable to wait until the 17th week and to inject 100 milligrams of Rivanol intra-amniotically--a procedure safer than evacuation from below at 14—16 weeks. In recent years, the use of prostaglandin and its derivatives to terminate both early and mid-trimester pregnancies are on clinical trial. Prostaglandin is most frequently used for abortions soon after delivery or cesarean section.

INCIDENCE OF INDUCED ABORTION

The incidence of induced abortion has been very high, especially in urban areas of the People's Republic of China. Table 1 shows the incidence of abortion in three recent population-based surveys. Each of the surveys, which represent either an administrative district or a metropolitan area in Xian, Shanghai, and Beijing cities, was conducted in 1981 and 1982. The rates of abortion appear similar in all three cities, but slightly higher in Xian and Beijing than Shanghai. The three samples indicate that nearly half of the respondents had experienced at least one abortion by the time of the interview. The annual rate of abortion in Beijing was 6.7 per 100 married women aged 20—49, and 4.8 per 100 women regardless of marital status. The total abortion rate was 1.9 per married woman, and 1.3 per woman. The abortion ratio in the most recent three years was 75 per 100 live births.

The high incidence of abortion in these three cities is still below the highest levels documented in other countries. Tietze (1983) shows that the rate of abortion per 100 women in Romania and Bulgaria was 8.8 and 7.0 respectively in 1979, and in Japan, 8.4 in 1975. The same document also shows that the world's highest recorded abortion rates per 100 women were 25.2 for Romania in the 1964—65 period, 22.0 for the USSR in 1965, and 13.8 for Japan in 1960. The highest abortion ratio per 100 live births reached 408 for Romania in 1965, followed by 275 in the USSR in 1965, and 197 in Japan in 1960.

Table 1

Data on Induced Abortion from Sample Surveys Conducted in Xian (1981),
Shanghai (1981), and Beijing (1982) Cities, People's Republic of China

Indicators of the Incidence of Induced Abortion	Sampling Surveys in Cities of:		
	Xian	Shanghai	Beijing
1. Proportion of respondents having had an induced abortion	45.9%	46.4%	44.8%
At least: once	28.7	34.4	31.2
two times	14.1	10.0	11.5
three or more	3.1	2.0	2.1
2. Annual Rate of Abortion* (Per 100 Women)			
Married Women	7.4	5.0	6.7
All Women	--	2.6	4.8
3. Total Abortion Rate* (Per Woman)			
Married Women	2.0	1.8	1.9
All Women	--	0.9	1.3
4. Abortion Ratio (Per 100 Live Births)			
1977-79	72	87	70
1980-81	123	84	--
1980-82	--	--	75
(Number of Respondents)**	(1,051)	(2,822)	(3,830)

* The rates are based on data for the year prior to the surveys conducted. Both Xian and Shanghai Surveys were conducted at the end of 1981, and the Beijing survey was conducted at the end of 1982, on a sampling basis. The three samples respectively represent 700,000 population in a district of Xian City, about 6 million population in Metro-Shanghai, and 764,000 population in a district of Beijing City respectively.
** Married women aged below 50 at time of interview.

Table 2 presents sociodemographic differentials in the rate of abortion in 1982 from the Beijing survey. Since an abortion is preconditioned by a pregnancy, the table shows both abortion and pregnancy rates. For all respondents, as shown in the first row of the table, there was an average of 6.7 abortions out of 15.4 pregnancies per 100 women. The youngest age group had the highest pregnancy rate but a relatively low rate of abortion because few pregnancies ended by abortion. Pregnancy rates decreased steadily with increasing age, and, except for the youngest age group, the abortion rate also decreased with increasing age of the woman. Of all childless women, 5.5 percent had an abortion in that year. Respondents with one prior live birth had the highest rate of abortion. Notice that a very high proportion of pregnancies of women with one or more prior live births were aborted. Respondents in the group of lowest education had very low abortion and pregnancy rates due to their old ages. Those who have the highest education had a lower abortion rate because of their low pregnancy rate. Among different occupational groups, the differentials in abortion rates were insignificant. However, officials and party cadres appeared to have a lower abortion rate because of a lower pregnancy rate.

Table 2
Abortion and Pregnancy Rates in 1982 by Characteristics of Respondent
Xi-Cheng District, Beijing City, 1982

Characteristics of Respondent (Currently Married (20-40)	Abortion Rate	Pregnancy Rate	Number of Respondents
Total	6.7%	15.4%	(3,783)*
Age: 20-24	7.8	48.8	(139)
25-29	16.9	43.2	(873)
30-34	9.3	15.0	(702)
35-39	4.1	4.6	(610)
40-44	0.7	0.7	(754)
45-49	0.0	0.0	(705)
Respondent's Number of Prior Live Births			
0	5.5	55.4	(630)
1	14.2	15.2	(1,284)
2	3.1	3.5	(1,093)
3+	0.4	0.4	(776)
Education			
Primary or less	1.2	1.9	(805)
Junior High	9.9	21.6	(1,694)
Senior High	6.7	23.9	(509)
College or Higher	5.5	10.6	(775)
Occupation			
Professional and Technical	7.3	14.1	(947)
Officials & Party Cadres	5.3	11.0	(432)
Commercial and Services	6.6	18.2	(697)
Industrial Workers	7.1	16.7	(1,627)
Others**	1.3	6.6	(80)

* Number of respondents at mid-year of 1982.
** Housewives, retirees, students, and farmers. Both abortion and pregnancy rates for this group are unreliable because of too few observations.

Table 3 presents sociodemographic characteristics of respondents having had an abortion by the year of last abortion performed in the Beijing Survey. To avoid bias of a retrospective survey toward young ages, we decided to disregard the first period, 1955–1972, and to compare the last two periods: 1973–79 and 1980–82, or before and after the one-child policy. Since the one-child policy was implemented in 1980–82, a greater proportion of respondents had their last abortion performed at a younger age, with fewer prior live births, belonged to the middle educated group, and were using the service of local hospitals or clinics.

Respondents who had an abortion were asked the reason for their last abortion. Since induced abortion has long been legalized, the topic appears to be less of a political, moral, and ethical issue as in some Western countries. Therefore, we regard respondents' answers to this question to be highly believable. Table 4 shows the percentage distribution of the most important reason for the last abortion by type of abortion and age, prior live births, and education of the woman. The reasons for abortion were ordered according to the degree of self-motivation: from being persuaded as being the least motivated to health reason as being the

Table 3

Percentage Distribution for Characteristics of Respondent Having
Last Abortion by the Year of Abortion Performed
Xi-Cheng District, Beijing City, 1982

Characteristics of Respondent with Abortion	Total	The Year of Last Abortion		
		1955-72*	73-79	80-82
Total Respondents	100.0%	100.0%	100.0%	100.0%
(Number of Respondents)	(1,713)	(547)	(602)	(564)
Age at Last Abortion				
19-24	6.2%	10.4%	3.7%	5.0%
25-29	41.3	45.0	31.6	48.0
30-39	33.1	35.3	33.7	30.3
40-49	19.4	9.3	31.1	16.7
Number of Live Births Prior to Abortion				
0	5.4	3.1	3.0	10.1
1	45.2	23.2	43.5	68.4
2	30.8	36.0	37.7	18.4
3+	18.6	37.7	15.8	3.0
Years of Schooling				
0	22.4	45.2	17.6	5.3
1-9	42.8	23.2	41.4	63.5
10+	34.8	31.6	41.0	31.2
Place Abortion Performed				
City Hospital	72.6	70.4	76.4	70.6
District Hospital	17.2	18.8	15.8	17.2
Local Hospital/Clinics	10.2	10.8	7.8	12.2

* Data on last abortions performed during this period should be disregarded, since this is observed too far back in time, and would involve a bias toward young ages because of the truncation of old respondents at time of last abortion.

most strongly motivated. The top row of the table shows that only 4.2 percent of total abortions were performed as a result of persuasion by officials responsible for the birth planning program, 23.3 percent to comply with the governmental policy of birth planning, 65.1 percent were abortions of either mistimed or unwanted pregnancies, and 7.4 percent were performed for protecting maternal health.

Classifying the distribution of the reason by calendar years of last abortion performed, the proportion performed because the woman was persuaded or because of policy compliance has greatly increased in recent years, especially after the one-child policy was enforced in 1980. The increase in the proportion performed because of policy compliance in the 1980–82 period was mostly accounted for by aborting the pregnancies occurring to couples who took a pledge to have only one child. In fact, the survey also revealed that virtually all (96%) one-child couples had taken a pledge to have one child and received a one-child certificate at the time of the survey. When classified by weeks gestation, the proportion performed for health reasons increased with length of gestation.

The pattern of respondents' age distribution is very similar to the pattern by respondents' parity. The older women, or women with higher parity, had a higher

Table 4
Percentage Distribution of Reasons for Last Abortion by Type
of Last Abortion or Woman, Xi-Cheng District, Beijing City, 1982

Characteristics of Last Abortion or Woman	Reason for Last Induced Abortion				Total	(N)**
	Being Persuaded (a)	Complied with Policy (b)	Unplanned Pregnancy (c)	Health Reasons (d)		
Total	4.2%	23.3%	65.1%	7.4%	100.0%	(1,713)
Year of Abortion						
1955-72	0.7	5.3	85.2	8.8	100.0	(547)
73-79	3.2	17.4	73.6	5.8	100.0	(602)
80-82	8.7	47.0	36.5	7.8	100.0	(564)
Weeks Gestation						
8 Weeks or Less	4.3	22.8	67.0	5.9	100.0	(1,007)
9 - 12 Weeks	4.5	24.9	63.2	7.3	100.0	(506)
13 - 16 Weeks	3.0	21.8	60.6	14.5	100.0	(165)
17 and More	2.9	20.0	57.1	20.0	100.0	(35)
Age at Abortion						
19-24	7.5	15.9	62.6	14.0	100.0	(107)
25-29	5.2	28.9	57.0	8.9	100.0	(707)
30-34	3.4	22.8	67.8	6.0	100.0	(567)
35-49	2.4	14.8	78.3	4.5	100.0	(332)
Prior Live Births						
0	5.4	10.9	37.0	46.7	100.0	(92)
1	7.2	38.1	48.0	6.7	100.0	(775)
2	1.3	15.0	80.1	3.6	100.0	(528)
3+	1.3	4.7	89.9	4.1	100.0	(318)
Years of Schooling						
0	2.1	10.2	81.2	6.5	100.0	(383)
1-9	5.9	35.6	51.9	6.7	100.0	(734)
10+	3.5	16.6	71.0	8.9	100.0	(596)

(a) The abortion was persuaded by officials who were responsible for the birth planning program.
(b) Those who voluntarily complied with the birth planning policy, or the one-child
policy after 1980, and those who have pledged and accepted an one-child family
certificate.
(c) Mistimed and unwanted pregnancies for reasons related to economy, housing,
employment, study, and other personal reasons.
(d) Due to bad health or advised by doctors to protect maternal health.

proportion of unplanned pregnancies and had a lower proportion of health reasons.
In terms of educational background, more women with mid-level education had
abortions because of being persuaded and policy compliance compared with the
other two groups.

PERIOD OF GESTATION

The period of gestation at which a pregnancy is terminated is an important
risk factor associated with induced abortion. Table 5 lists the percentage distribu-

Table 5
Percentage Distribution of Abortions by Weeks Gestation
for Selected Area and Countries

	Weeks Gestation			
	11 Weeks or Less	12-14 Weeks	16 Weeks or More	Total
Beijing City, People's Republic of China:				
a. City Hospital:				
1982	87.0%	5.5%	7.5%	100.0%
1983	89.7	4.2	6.1	100.0
1984	89.8	5.2	4.9	100.0

	8 weeks or less	9-12 weeks	13-16 weeks	17 weeks or more	Total
b. District Hosp., 1980-82:	82.6%	15.2%	2.2%	0.0%	100.0%
c. Regional Survey, 1982:	58.8	29.5	9.6	2.1	100.0
United States, 1980:	51.7	38.3	5.2	4.8	100.0
New York State, 1980:					
Resident	51.7	37.4	6.8	4.1	100.0
Nonresident	39.3	26.7	9.3	24.7	100.0
England & Wales, 1980:					
Resident	24.7	57.4	13.1	4.8	100.0
Nonresident	20.4	47.4	20.9	11.3	100.0
Canada, 1980:	24.6	61.4	10.4	3.6	100.0
Sweden, 1980:	38.0	56.9	3.6	1.5	100.0
Denmark, 1980:	37.7	59.5	1.4	1.4	100.0
Hungary, 1980:	67.1	31.9	0.6	0.4	100.0
Czechoslovakia, 1980:	55.7	43.8	0.4	0.1	100.0
Japan, 1978:	----- 95.5 -----		----- 4.5 -----		100.0
India, 1978/79:	----- 83.4 -----		----- 16.6 -----		100.0

a. The First Affiliated Hospital of Beijing Medical University.
b. One of District Hospitals in Tung-Cheng District, Beijing City.
c. Based on a sampling survey conducted in Xi-Cheng District, Beijing City.
Note: Except for the People's Republic of China, data shown in this table were excerpted from: Tietze, C., "Induced Abortion: A World Review, 1983," Table 13, 66-69.

tion of weeks gestation at abortion from the reports of two clinic-based studies conducted in hospitals and a population-based survey carried out in a district of Beijing City, as well as the statistics of selected countries. Among the three Beijing reports, the city hospital and the regional (district) survey indicated a much higher proportion of later mid-trimester abortions than that of the district hospital. Since the city hospital is better equipped for high-risk cases, it has performed more late gestation abortions. The report of the regional survey, however, involved higher proportions of later mid-trimester abortions performed in early years, which will be discussed in the next table. Compared with other countries, the proportions of late mid-trimester abortions of the three Beijing studies were not the lowest, but they were lower than those of New York State, England and Wales, Canada, and India.

Table 6 shows the differentials in proportion of last abortions performed after 12 weeks gestation by the year of abortion and characteristics of respondent from the Beijing survey. Of all respondents having had an abortion, 11.7 percent had their abortions performed after 12 weeks gestation, or during the mid-trimester pregnancy. Comparing the years during which the abortions were performed, there is a downward trend in the proportion of mid-trimester abortions. For instance, mid-trimester abortion dropped from 13.9 percent in 1955—72 to 11.3 percent in 1973—79, and further dropped to 10.0 percent in 1980—82. In terms of reasons for having the last abortion, being persuaded had the lowest, while health reasons represented the highest proportion for mid-trimester abortion. Among different age groups, the proportions were almost identical. Respondents without live births had mid-trimester abortions for health reasons which are greatly associated with late abortion. In terms of education, those women with no education at all were much more likely to have late abortion than the other two higher education groups. Finally, considering occupation, the incidence of mid-trimester abortion appeared to be the lowest for the officials, and, in contrast, the highest for commercial and service workers.

SHORT-TERM COMPLICATIONS

The rate of short-term complication associated with induced abortion in urban People's Republic of China has been as low as those of developed countries, even though almost all abortions were performed by paramedics on an outpatient basis. Table 7 shows the reports of symptoms by respondents in the Beijing survey. Since they are responses to questions by interviewers without medical background, rather than the diagnosis of medical professionals, the reliability of data should be carefully assessed and interpreted. The 1.4 percent of women being hospitalized with major symptoms, such as bleeding, infection, and abdominal pain, may be related to abortion complication. However, some of these symptoms may not have been associated with the procedure if the pregnancies were terminated for health reasons and the hospitalization could have resulted for reasons other than the abortion. The report by 4.6 percent of women of major symptoms without hospitalization and 13.0 percent of minor symptoms may also be less likely to have been associated with abortion complications.

Table 8 presents the rates of major complications associated with the procedure based on the clinical reports of two hospitals in Beijing City. Although the city hospital dealt with more high risk patients, it reported 0.3 percent had major complications, compared with a higher 0.5 percent reported by the district hospital. Nevertheless, these two rates appear to be much lower than the 1.4 percent who reported major symptoms with hospitalization in the population-based survey presented in the previous table. Most importantly, the rates of complication from either the clinical reports or the survey conducted in Beijing are within the range of the rates of studies conducted in other developed countries as shown in the table. Table 9 further compares the rates of specific symptoms of the two clinical studies and the sampling survey in Beijing with the studies conducted in other developed countries. Again, the three Chinese studies did not identify any complication substantially different from other studies.

CONCLUSIONS

More than 30 years of legalized induced abortion have not only relieved numerous couples from the burden of mistimed and unwanted pregnancies but have played an important role in lowering the level of fertility in urban People's Republic of China. The Chinese Government and medical profession have both repeat-

Table 6
Proportion of Abortions Performed after 12 Weeks Gestation by Characteristics of Respondent, Xi-Cheng District, Beijing City, 1982

Characteristics of Respondent at Last Abortion	Percent of Abortion Performed after 12 Weeks Gestation	Number of Abortions
All Respondents	11.7%	(1,713)
Year of Last Abortion		
1955-72	13.9	(547)
73-79	11.3	(602)
80-82	10.0	(564)
Reason for Last Abortion		
Being Persuaded	8.3	(92)
Policy Compliance	10.8	(399)
Unplanned Pregnancy	10.8	(1,115)
Health Reasons	24.4	(127)
Age at Last Abortion		
19-29	11.9	(814)
30-34	11.5	(567)
35-49	11.5	(332)
Number of Live Births Prior to Last Abortion		
0	25.0	(92)
1	10.3	(775)
2+	11.5	(846)
Years of Schooling		
0	15.2	(383)
1-9	9.8	(734)
10+	11.8	(596)
Occupation of Respondent		
Professional and Technical	11.9	(446)
Officials & Party Cadres	6.7	(210)
Commercial and Services	14.8	(298)
Industrial Workers	11.7	(725)
Others*	11.8	(34)

* Housewives, retirees, students, and farmers.

edly emphasized that abortion is a remedial measure for contraceptive failure but should not be used as a method of contraception. Therefore, to minimize the incidence of abortion, efforts should be made to increase the prevalence and improve the use-effectiveness of contraception. In addition to increasing the popularity of family planning education, more research to improve the existing contraceptives and to find new methods to meet the special needs of our country is deemed necessary to meet these objectives.

Results of our studies indicate that the abortions involved very little risk of short-term complications in spite of the fact that most of the procedures were performed by paramedics on an outpatient basis. The morbidity rate of those legal abortions has been kept much lower than what can be expected from illegal abortions performed by non-professionals. This was mainly attributed to strict adher-

Table 7
Percentage of Women Having Symptoms with Last Abortion
Xi-Cheng District, Beijing City, 1982

Symptoms	Percentage	
Major, Hospitalized	1.4	
Bleeding		0.7
Infection		0.6
Abdominal Pain		0.1
Major, Not Hospitalized	4.6	
Bleeding		1.9
Infection		1.5
Abdominal Pain		1.2
Minor	13.0	
Low Back Pain & Discomfort		6.9
Dizziness and Nausea		2.9
Malaise		1.9
Menstrual Irregularity		1.3
No Complaints	81.0	
Total	100.0	
(Women having Abortions)	(1,713)	

Note: For those who had multiple symptoms, only the symptom on the top of the hierarchical order as shown in the table was counted.
Data Source: Chen, Y. D., et al., "Short-term complication associated with induced in Beijing City, China," unpublished.

ence to quality control regulations and observance of operating protocol in the process of the procedure.

In contrast to our knowledge in urban areas, very little is known about the practice and health problems associated with induced abortion in rural areas, where the great majority of the Chinese population resides. Therefore, large-scale surveillance programs and well-designed clinical studies are to be conducted not only in urban areas, but also in rural villages, to bring about further improvement of the health of Chinese women.

Table 8
Rates of Major Complications Associated with Induced Abortion Based on Studies Conducted in Beijing City and Selected Countries

Studies	% of Women Having Major Complication	Remarks
Beijing City, People's Republic of China:		
a. City Hospital (1982)	0.3%	Suction and curettage; dilatation and evacuation.
b. District Hospital (1980-82)	0.5	Mostly by suction and curettage by paramedics on an outpatient basis.
c. Regional Survey, 1982		
All with major symptoms:	6.0	Same as above.
Only being hospitalized:	1.4	
United States, 1970-78	0.1-0.7	Suction and curettage.
United States, 1972-75	0.3	Suction and curettage, adolescent.
New York State, 1980	1.2	Methods unspecified.
Czechoslovakia, 1980	0.2	" "
England & Wales, 1980	0.9	" "
German Fed. Rep., 1980	2.4	" "
Canada, 1980	2.4	" "
Denmark, 1980	3.9	" "

a. The First Affiliated Hospital of Beijing Medical University.
b. One of District Hospitals in Tung-Cheng District, Beijing City.
c. Based on a sampling survey conducted in Xi-Cheng District, Beijing City.
Data Source: Except data from the City and District hospitals, other figures shown in this table were duplicated from: Chen, Y. D., et al., "Short-term complication associated with induced in Beijing City, China," unpublished.

REFERENCES

Cates, W. Adolescent abortions in the United States. Journal of Adolescent Health Care 1:18, 1980.
Cates, W., Grimes, D. A. Morbidity and mortality of abortion in the United States. In J. E. Hodgson, ed., Abortion and Sterilization, p. 155. Academic Press, London, 1981.
Chen, C. H. C. Short-term complications associated with induced abortion in Beijing City, unpublished, 1986.
Faundes, A., Luukkainen, T. Health and family planning services in China. Studies in Family Planning, 3:173 (Supplement), 1972.
Feng, Z. H., Chen, C. H. C. Induced abortion in Xian City, China. International Family Planning Perspectives 9:81, 1983.
Gao, E. S., Chen, C. H. C., Rochat, R. W. Epidemiology of pregnancy outcome in Shanghai City, The People's Republic of China. Paper presented at the

Table 9
Specific Symptoms Associated with Abortion for Beijing Studies and
Comparative Complications with Suction and Curettage Procedure
Performed at 12 Weeks or Less Gestation for Selected Studies

Areas and Countries of Studies	Complication Rate per 100 Procedures				Number of Patients
	Uterine Hemorrhage	Pelvic Infection	Cervical Injury	Uterine Perforation	
Beijing City, People's Republic of China:					
a. City Hosp., 1982	0.009*	0.0	0.0	0.036	(9,860)
b. Dist. Hosp., 1980–82	0.060*	0.0	NS	0.030	(10,852)
c. Region. Survey, 1982	0.7**	0.6**	NA	NA	(1,713)
Beric et al., 1971	3.4	0.3	0.1	0.1	(6,445)
Nathanson, 1972	0.2	1.5	NS	0.1	(26,000)
Stewart et al., 1972	4.9	1.2	NS	0.7	(3,482)
Walton, 1972	0.1	NS	0.2	0.2	(4,222)
Tietze et al., 1972	1.0	0.6	0.9	0.3	(47,618)
Edelman et al., 1974	1.3	2.0	0.8	0.2	(2,972)
Hodgson, 1975	0.05	0.7	0.01	0.1	(20,248)
Wulff et al., 1977	0.3	0.1	0.1	0.2	(16,410)
Bozorgi, 1977	0.2	0.1	0.2	0.02	(10,890)
Andolscek et al., 1977	0.1	2.2	0.1	0.1	(4,470)
Smith et al., 1978	1.0	0.8	1.6	0.1	(13,252)
Cates et al., 1979	0.4	0.7	1.0	0.2	(54,155)

a. The First Affiliated Hospital of Beijing Medical University. This study also detected 0.19 and 0.03 percent of incomplete abortion and uterine adhesion respectively.

b. One of District Hospitals in Tung-Cheng District, Beijing City. This study also detected 0.13 and 0.29 percent of incomplete abortion and uterine adhesion respectively.

c. Based on a sampling survey conducted in Xi-Cheng District, Beijing City.

* More than 200 ml of blood loss.

** Being hospitalized because of the symptom.

NA = Not Available.

NS = Not Stated.

Data Source: Except for data from Beijing City, this table was duplicated from "Morbidity and mortality of abortion in the United States," Table 3, p. 162, in Abortion and Sterilization, J. E. Hodgson, ed., Academic Press, London, 1981.

Annual Meeting of American Public Health Association, Washington, DC, Nov. 17–21, 1985.

Grimes, D. A., Schultz, K. F., Cates, W., et al. The Joint Program for the Study of Abortion/CDC: a preliminary report. In W. Hern, B. Andrikopoulos, Abortion in the Seventies. National Abortion Federation, New York, 1977.

Tietze, C. Induced Abortion: A World Review 1983. The Population Council, New York, 1983.

Wang, S. X., et al. Proximate determinants of fertility in Beijing City, The People's Republic of China. Studies in Family Planning, the Population Council, New York (in press).

MEDICAL PRACTICE AFTER LEGALIZATION OF ABORTION: BANGLADESH

Halida H. Akhter

The World Bank
Population, Health and Nutrition
Washington, D.C.

HISTORICAL DEVELOPMENT OF ABORTION POLICY AND LEGAL STATUS OF ABORTION

The population of Bangladesh is now around 100 million with an estimated growth rate of 2.6 percent annually. Population density is one of the highest in the world at more than 600 persons per square km. The age structure of the population gives a high dependency ratio (93 percent) with 45 percent of the population below 15 years. Total fertility rate remains high, estimated at 5.8 in 1985. Extended breastfeeding practice leads to relatively long birth intervals of approximately 3 years. Early marriage is still the norm. More than 50 percent of women get married by the age of 16 (1981). Health status of the population is unacceptably low with an estimated infant mortality of 125/1000 live births and maternal mortality of 5.7/1000 live births (1975). At least a quarter of this high maternal mortality is due to complications of indigenously induced abortions.

Under the Bangladesh Penal Code of 1860, induced abortion is permitted only to save the life of the mother. In 1972, the law was waived for women raped during the War of Liberation. Abortions were performed in a few district hospitals under the guidance of expert teams from Bangladesh, India, the United Kingdom, and the United States. In 1976, legalization of first-trimester abortion on broad medical and social grounds was proposed, but legislative action was not taken.

The government encouraged the introduction of menstrual regulation (MR) services in a few isolated family planning clinics in 1974. In 1978, the Pathfinder Fund initiated a MR training and services program in seven government medical colleges and two government district hospitals. Training was given to government doctors and paramedics (Family Welfare Visitors, FWVs) and a few private doctors. In 1979, the government included MR in the national family planning program and encouraged doctors and paramedics to provide MR services in all government hospitals, health and family planning complexes (BPCFPD Memo, May & December 1979). Citing a Law Institute paper, the government noted that MR is not regulated by the Penal Code, since pregnancy is difficult or impossible to prove. Rather, MR is said to be an "interim method of establishing nonpregnancy for a woman at risk of being pregnant, whether or not she actually is pregnant (Bangladesh Institute of Law and International Affairs, 1979).

By 1984, about 2,100 doctors (government and private) and 2,200 government FWVs had been trained in MR (Table 1). Reported MR procedures have risen from 4,000 in 1975-76 to 50-60,000 per year in 1983-84 (Table 2), but the actual number

Table 1: Distribution of Trained Physicians and Paramedics (FWV*)
in Eleven MR Training Centers

MR Training Centers	Year MR Training Started	Total Trained up to 1984	
		Doctor	FWV
Mohammadpur Fertility Services and Training Centre, Dhaka	1975	89	698
Dhaka Medical College Hospital	1979	628	--
Sir Salimullah Medical College Hospital	1979	499	46
Chittagong Medical College Hospital	1979	164	195
Rangpur Medical College Hospital	1980	126	193
Sher-e-Bangla Medical College Hospital, Barisal	1981	150	163
Sylhet Medical College Hospital	1981	152	146
Mymensingh Medical College Hospital	1981	155	236
Pabna Sadar Hospital	1981	87	188
Khulna Sadar Hospital	1981	94	196
Bangladesh Women's Health Coalition clinics	1982	+	131
Total		2,144	2,192

Source: Data compiled by Bangladesh Association for Prevention of Septic Abortion (BAPSA), published in their Quarterly MR Newsletter, May 1985.
* Family Welfare visitors, a paramedic group.
+ Do not train doctors.

may be much higher. Social stigma attached to MR and abortion may inhibit reporting and the reporting system is, in any case, poor. It may also be assumed that a large number of MRs are performed in private practice and are not reported. Trained providers are dispersed throughout the country, primarily in government health complexes and centers at various administrative levels.

Because records have not been kept, the exact number and location of trained providers are not known. A study involving 376 physicians in 173 health complexes, 44 hospitals, and 26 non-hospital centers including family planning centers observed that about half provide pregnancy termination services, menstrual regulation services, and referral for pregnancy termination services (Table 3) (Rosenberg, 1981).

The government provides considerable support in the form of clinic space, salaries, and equipment for MR training and services. Until 1983, external funds were available from USAID, the Pathfinder Fund, and the Population Crisis Committee. Due to the U.S. government stance on abortion, in 1983-84 almost all nongovernment programs stopped providing MR services in order to protect their USAID funds. At present only three programs, two quasi-government and one nongovernment, train government health personnel (doctors and FWVs) in the MR

Table 2: Menstrual Regulation Procedures,
Bangladesh, 1975–1984.

Year	Number of MRs performed
1975-76	4,408
1976-77	6,687
1977-78	6,135
1978-79	4,412
1979-80	10,479
1980-81	28,041
1981-82	42,427
1982-83	58,579
1983-84	56,728

Source: Population Control Bulletin.
* The performance statistics on MR services are collected as a part of family planning and MCH service by Management Information System (MIS) unit of the Directorate of Population Control.

Table 3: Reproductive Services Provided by Physician Respondents in Past Year: Abortion Attitude Survey, Bangladesh, 1978-79
(n=376)

Type of Services	Percent providing service*
One or more services below	92.0
Delivery	82.1
Referral for pregnancy termination	45.2
Pregnancy termination (abortion at 12 or more weeks of gestation)	45.2
Menstrual regulation (abortion up to 12 weeks of gestation)	31.6
IUD insertion	10.9

Source: Rosenberg et al. "Attitudes of Rural Bangladesh Physicians towards Abortion. Studies in Family Planning, Vol. 12, No. 8/9, August/September 1981, pp. 318–321.
aTotals do not add to 100 because of multiple responses.

procedure. The government in its Third Five-Year Plan (1985–1990) proposes to extend MR facilities in terms of trained staff and equipment to rural-level health complexes throughout the country.

LEGAL STATUS OF ABORTION

Efforts were made to legalize first-trimester abortion on broad medical and social grounds as early as 1976 in the Bangladesh National Population Policy (Choudhury and Susan, 1975). As of 1985, this has not been implemented and restrictive legislation remains in effect (Al-Qaliqili, 1977). Nevertheless, a memorandum from the Population Control and Family Planning Division (PCFPD) states categorically that "menstrual regulation" (MR) is one of the methods used in the national family planning program. The memorandum quotes a report from the Institute of Law (1979) to the effect that MR does not come under the provision of penal code Section 312 in regard to abortion because pregnancy cannot be established. The Institute of Law report (1979) also mentioned:

> Moreover, many Family Planning Clinics are carrying out the post-contraceptive method of "Menstrual Regulation" as a means of birth control which does not come under section 312 of the Penal Code. Under statutory scheme, pregnancy is an essential element of the crime of abortion, but the use of menstrual regulations makes it virtually impossible for the prosecutor to meet the required proof. In our country menstrual regulation (MR) is being carried out till the tenth week following a missed menstrual period, and after that patients are referred as abortion cases. MR is now recognised as an interim method of establishing non-pregnancy for the woman who is at risk of being pregnant. Whether or not she is, in fact, pregnant is no longer an issue.

The Population Control and Family Planning circular of May 1979 states that MR is included in the official policy and necessary logistic support for MR services and training will be provided by the Division. Another PCFPD memorandum in 1980 permits the performance of MR by an MR-trained registered medical practitioner and any Family Welfare Visitor (FWV, a paramedic) who has specific training in MR (BPCFPD Memo, 1980). It also specifies that an FWV should perform MR only up to eight weeks from last menstrual period, i.e., four weeks from missed menstrual period, under the supervision of a physician. Any case with longer duration must be referred to a trained doctor. In many government-supported clinics the procedure is performed by paramedics (Bhatia and Ruzicka, 1978). The Second Five-Year Plan released in 1980 envisaged that menstrual regulation facilities will be provided through the family planning clinics, welfare centers, all health centers, and hospitals (Akhter and Rider, 1984).

MR TRAINING: DOCTORS AND PARAMEDICS

It is difficult to say how many persons should be trained and given equipment for menstrual regulation. The draft Third Five-Year Plan (1985–1990) proposes to extend MR facilities (trained staff and equipment) to "upazila" (county) level health complexes, of which there are 450. Over and above the existing 4,000 trained providers, the draft plan proposed training 1,000 more doctors and 600 more FWVs. The doctors' training estimate is reasonable and, in our review, is the maximum number needed. However, it is important to train all 2,500 FWVs who have not yet been trained as they are always posted at the local level, and they are all women and thus more likely to be acceptable to women seeking MR (most doctors are men). Equally important in our judgment is refresher training for those already trained, and careful supervision and follow-up of providers. A summary of estimated training needs is given in Table 4. Table 5 provides data on the training capacity per year of the three training centers.

Criteria have been set for a standardized MR training curriculum for both doctors and FWVs. Training is given for a minimum of one, but preferably (and usually) two weeks. Each trainee performs at least 20 pelvic examinations to estimate length of gestation, observes ten MR procedures, and performs at least ten. Trainees are instructed to refer women whose pregnancies are estimated to be more than 8 weeks to other hospital facilities. The training also covers recognition and management of gynecological complications, sterile technique, care and maintenance of equipment, clinic management, and contraceptive counseling for MR clients. The three training programs operate "model" family planning services to ensure that trainees recognize the importance, not simply of the MR procedure, but also of follow-up care and contraceptive counseling to encourage women to avoid repeat MR procedures.

Table 4: New and Refresher Training Required, 1985–90

	Doctors		FWVs	
	Required 1985-90	Proposed for FF Funding	Required 1985-90	Proposed For FF Funding
New	1,000	(808)	2,500[a]	(988)[c]
Refresher[a]	2,000	(192)	2,700	(588)

[a]Assumes all providers should have refresher training but that only two thirds can be identified and deputed for training. The number includes both those trained to date and those proposed for training 1985-90.

[b]Government proposes only 600 in the draft Third Five-Year Plan.

[c]Includes 100 student FWVs as well as in-service FWVs.

Table 5: M.R. Training Capacity per Year

		New		Refresher		Number of
Organization	Total	FWV	Doctor	FWV	Doctor	Centers
MRTSP	864	384	384	48	48	9 (new) 2 (refresher)
MFSTC	224	60	20	96	48	1
BWHC	135	35[a]	--	100	--	4
	1,223	479	404	244	96	

[a]These are student FWVs.

Finally, research and documentation are needed not only to strengthen the training and service programs but also to build the case for continuing provision of MR services, especially by the government. The Measham and Rochat estimates of induced abortions per year and of mortality and morbidity rates need to be updated. More should be known about the attitudes of village health workers and traditional practitioners toward abortion. Outreach techniques should be developed to persuade women to seek early, medically supervised services rather than resort to clandestine procedures. Ultimately, the law should be further liberalized, but it is reasonable as it stands and to raise the issue now could result in regressive revision.

QUALITY OF CARE

Since the inception of MR services in Bangladesh, both physicians and paramedics are being trained to provide MR services. Initially, in a few small clinics, paramedics used to do MR procedures under direct supervision of physicians. Now they provide MR more or less independently in their respective place of work and private clinics. However, they are expected to keep good linkage with the doctors for supervision and for the referral of complicated cases. After MR training the trainees return to their respective place of posting. Although they are expected to report their MR performances, usually they do not report. However, efforts are currently being made to improve the reporting system and to encourage providers to report. This reporting will serve the purpose of surveillance and will provide information on acceptability, safety, and quality of MR service provided by the physicians as well as the paramedics.

One small evaluation of MR training and services programs in Bangladesh studied 372 women obtaining MR at the centers of 40 physicians and 48 paramedics during a 3-month period starting in December 1981. Cluster samples of the clinics of trained physicians and paramedics were selected from five districts which represented four administrative divisions of the country. Immediate MR complication rate was not significantly different between the clients of physicians (6 percent) and paramedics (7.3 percent). No major life-threatening immediate complications were reported in either group (Measham, 1981). Demographic characteristics associated with complications, e.g., age, parity, and education, were not significantly different in the two groups. Over 80 percent of the clients of each group expressed satisfaction with short waiting time, short duration of the procedure, dealings of the clinic personnel, and the procedure being less expensive than they expected. Slightly more than one-third of each group found the procedure painful. This study reported higher febrile morbidity among the paramedics' clients. This may be due to difference in the sterile technique used for the procedure and the instruments, duration of the procedure, and use of prophylactic antibiotics. Another factor that might have contributed to higher febrile morbidity is that paramedics were more likely than the physicians to provide clients with IUDs. However, since the study lacked data to evaluate contribution of these factors, more studies should be done to evaluate the safety of the procedures in remote rural areas.

FUTURE NEEDS

For the year 1978, Rochat (1981) and other Bangladeshi researchers estimated that at least 800,000 induced abortions occur every year in Bangladesh and that 25 percent of maternal mortality is due to induced abortion. The estimate has since been confirmed by smaller studies (BPCFPD Memo, 1979) and the consensus is that at least 8,000 women die every year from induced abortion. In addition, an unknown, but undoubtedly very large number of women suffer severe morbidity including sterility.

In an interview of seven selected indigenous abortion practitioners in rural Bangladesh, the practitioners gave a wide range of statistics on the number of abortions they perform (Islam, 1981). The performance ranged from a minimum of 3 to 4 cases in 8 or 9 years of the practitioner's career to a maximum of 1,000 induced abortions. Some perform several cases per month; one of them had performed 120 to 150 cases during the previous 3 years; others' performance ranged from 50 to 60 or 200–300 cases.

Although over the last several years menstrual regulation has been increasingly made available, in rural areas the service is not adequate to deal with the number of unwanted pregnancies. Clandestine abortions are still being practiced, especially in rural areas. In a health worker survey it was found that nearly half of the complicated abortions were induced by inserting such objects as sticks or roots into the uterus, or by vigorous physical activities. The most common practice was to insert a tree root into the uterus and leave it in place until an abortion or complications ensued. Insertion of foreign bodies was about five times as common as the use of oral preparations, the next most common method used (Jabeen, 1978).

If we compare the reports of 60,000 MRs performed annually in the country with the Rochat estimate of 800,000 abortions per year, it seems many more women need safe MR procedures to deal with their unwanted pregnancies. Comparing characteristics of women who received MR with those who were hospitalized for serious abortion complications one can observe that MR clients are higher educated, younger, of low parity, and in large proportion urban dwellers. It appears that to whatever extent MR service is available, it is not reaching high parity, less educated rural poor women. To meet with the demand of MR in rural areas, there must be MR training and retraining of the medical and paramedical personnel to deliver services safely. More government support is needed to extend safe MR services in rural areas by increasing training facilities and the quality of training. The law should be further liberalized but it is not unreasonable as it stands. Raising the issue at this time may result in regressive revision.

REFERENCES/BIBLIOGRAPHY

Ahmad, R. Attitude towards induced abortion in Bangladesh. Quarterly Journal of the Bangladesh Institute of Development Studies 7(4), Autumn 1979.

Ahmed, T., Kabir, M. A retrospective study on complications in MR--An investigation of socio-cultural causes. Contraceptive Practice in Bangladesh: Safety Issues: Report of Multi-Institutional Contraceptive Safety Research Program, Dhaka, December 1984.

Akhter, H. H., Rider, R. V. Menstrual regulation versus contraception in Bangladesh: Characteristicts of the acceptors Part 1. Studies in Family Planning 14(12)(December):318, 1983.

Akhter, H. H., Rider, R. V. Continuation of contraception following menstrual regulation--A Bangladesh experience. Journal of Biosocial Science 16:137, 1984a.

Akhter, H. H., Rider, R. V. Menstrual regulation and contraception in Bangladesh: Competing or complementary? International Journal of Gynaecology & Obstetrics 22:137, 1984b.

Al-Qaliqili, Sheikh Abdullah (the Grand Mufti of Jordon). Fatwa: Family planning in Islam. In Islam and Family Planning. Directorate of Population Control and Family Planning, Government of the Peoples Republic of Bangladesh, Dhaka, 1977.

Bangladesh Fertility Survey 1975–1976. Ministry of Health and Population Control, Population Control and Family Planning Division, Government of the Peoples Republic of Bangladesh, First Report, Dhaka, 1978.

Bangladesh Institute of Law and International Affairs. Chapter II--Abortion. In Dhaka Report on Legal Aspects of Population Planning in Bangladesh, p. 31, 1979.

Bangladesh Planning Commission. The second five-year plan, Ministry of Planning, Paragragh XVII/87, Dhaka, 1980.

Bangladesh Population Control and Family Planning Division. Bangladesh National Population Policy. Government of People's Republic of Bangladesh, Dhaka, 1976.

Bangladesh Population Control and Family Planning Division. Circular No. FP/Misc-26/79/278 (600), Government of People's Republic of Bangladesh, May 31, 1979.

Bangladesh Population Control and Family Planning Division Memo No. 5-14/MCH-FP/Trg/79, Government of People's Republic of Bangladesh, December 8, 1979.

Bangladesh Population Control and Family Planning Division. Memo No. 5-14/MCH-FP/80, 1980.

Begum, S. F., Khan, A. R., Jahan, S. A study of 1,003 induced and spontaneous abortion patients treated at Dhaka Medical College. Bangladesh Technical Report No. 8, Bangladesh Fertility Research Program, Aug.–Oct. 1978.

Bhatia, S., Ruzicka, L. T. Menstrual regulation clients in a village-based family planning programme. Journal of Biosocial Science 1:12, 1980.

Bhuiyan, N., Begum, R., Begum, S. Characteristics of abortion cases admitted in Chittagong Medical College Hospital in 1978. Technical Report No. 33, November 1979.

Bichitra Newspaper, Dhaka, August 1977.

Chaudhury, R. H. Attitude of some elites towards introduction of abortion as a method of family planning in Bangladesh. Quarterly Journal of the Bangladesh Institute of Development Studies 3(4), October 1975.

Chaudhury, R. H. Attitudes towards legalization of abortion among a cross-section of women in metropolitan Dacca. Journal of Biosocial Science 12:417, 1980.

Chen, L. C., Gesche, M. C., Ahmed, S. Maternal mortality in rural Bangladesh. Studies in Family Planning 5:331, 1975.

Choudhury, Zaffrullah and Susan. Abortion in Bangladesh. The Bangladesh Times, Dhaka, May 3 and 5, 1975.

Hassan, S. Should abortion be legalized? Desperate women seek quack's help. The Bangladesh Times, December 13-14, Dhaka, 1976.

Islam, S. Indigenous abortion practitioners in rural Bangladesh. Women for Women: A Research Study Group, Dhaka, 1981.

Jabeen, S. Maternal mortality in Sir Salimullah Medical College (Mitford Hospital) from October 1976 to September 1978. Magazine '77, Sir Salimullah Medical College 1978:31, 1978.

Jabeen, S., Nazmul, S., Ahmed, G. A study of the abortion-related cases admitted in Sir Salimullah Medical College Hospital, Dhaka. Technical Report No. 35, November 1979.

Khan, A. R., Begum, S. F., Covington, D. L., et al. Risks and cost of illegally induced abortion in Bangladesh. Journal of Biosocial Science 16(1):89, 1984.

Measham, A. R., Obaidullah, M., Rosenberg, M. J. Complications from induced abortion in Bangladesh related to types of practitioners and methods, and impact on morbidity. Lancet, p. 199, January 1981.

Rochat, R. W., Jabeen, S., Rosenberg, M. J. Maternal and abortion related deaths in Bangladesh, 1978-79, International Journal of Gynaecology and Obstetrics 19:155, 1981.

Rosenberg, M. J., Rochat, R. W., Jabeen, S., et al. Attitudes of rural Bangladesh physicians toward abortion. Studies in Family Planning 12:318, 1981.

Waliullah, S., Al-Sabir, Ahmed. A study on menstrual regulation programme in two clinics. In Contraceptive Practice in Bangladesh: Safety issues. Report of Multi-Institutional Contraceptive Safety Research Program, Dhaka, December 1984.

SOME LESSONS FROM THE UNITED STATES EXPERIENCE WITH LEGAL ABORTION

P. G. Stubblefield

Chief of Obstetrics and Gynecology
Mount Auburn Hospital, Cambridge, Mass.
Associate Professor of Obstetrics and Gynecology
The Harvard Medical School
Boston, Mass., U.S.A.

THE NEW INSTITUTION

A decision of the U.S. Supreme Court made abortion legal throughout the U.S.A. in 1973 (Roe v. Wade, 1973). Prior to this time, only a few states, most notably New York, allowed legal abortion with few restrictions. In most states, legal abortions were limited to those women who could convince panels of physicians that their physical or mental illness was severe. In consequence, many illegal abortions were still performed (Legge, 1985).

The Court's decision in 1973 made abortion legal, but it did not make it universally available. Hospitals were not prepared to meet the need for large numbers of these procedures, and many had no interest in serving these women. A new institution was created to meet this need: the freestanding specialty abortion clinic. The clinic model which was developed and refined in New York City, Washington, D.C., and several other major cities, represented a new way to organize, finance, and deliver services to large numbers of clients at low cost. Components of the service were free pregnancy tests on a walk-in basis, and clinic operating hours on the weekend to make the service easily available for working women. Lay women were trained in a new profession, abortion counselors, ready to help with the psychological distress of the unwanted pregnancy. The complete surgical abortion service was provided by physicians who performed many abortions at each session, thereby becoming truly proficient and allowing reduced cost. The vacuum curettage technique was used from the outset, generally with local anesthesia. All relevant laboratory tests, Rh immune globulin for Rh negative women, contraceptive advice and services, and follow-up care of any complications were all provided as part of the same fee. Usually the counseling and abortion services were provided within the space of half a day. The cost was initially low and, corrected for inflation, costs are even less today. The opponents of legal abortion accuse the clinics of profiteering, but in fact a first-trimester abortion in a U.S. clinic costs markedly less than the smallest of hospital services and represents a true bargain in health care.

Since the abortion clinics began outside of the usual health care system, there was need for a national organization, and one has been created, the National Abortion Federation (NAF). This private organization, located in Washington, D.C., provides through its annual conventions and regional conferences a national forum for the sharing of experiences and solutions to common problems. The National Abortion Federation has developed written standards for the provision of abortion services that have been widely adopted. Presently more than half of U.S. abortions are performed in NAF member clinics.

UTILIZATION OF LEGAL ABORTION

The numbers of legal abortions rapidly increased from 1973 to level off at about 1.6 million per year, the current number. This increase caused those opposed to legal abortion to allege that abortion was replacing contraception. The more likely reality is that legal abortions have replaced procedures that formerly would have been done illegally and not reported. In addition, the number of women in the fertile years has increased since 1973, and young women are sexually active at an earlier age than they were in the past. Hence, in 1985 there are more women at risk for pregnancy than in 1973. National abortion ratios make a very telling point as to who uses abortion. The overall U.S. ratio of abortions to live births is 325/1000. For adolescents, the ratio is 2000/1000. For unmarried women, the ratio is 1600/1000, but for married women the ratio is only 100/1000 (Centers for Disease Control, 1979). Clearly, women are deciding to continue pregnancy when they themselves are married, no longer adolescents, and able to nurture a child.

We have detailed knowledge about legal abortion in the U.S. because of the Joint Program for the Study of Abortion (JPSA), a work begun by Christopher Tietze and Sarah Lewit. Tietze and Lewit obtained data from many hospitals and clinics using detailed questionnaires with standard coding of patient factors, procedures, and complications (Tietze and Lewit, 1972). JPSA was continued by the Centers for Disease Control (CDC) and complemented their epidemiologic surveillance of abortion. These studies provided the basis for more than 100 scientific articles on abortion written by the CDC scientists. Sadly, this important scholarship has largely come to a close during the administration of President Reagan, well known for its anti-legal-abortion bias. Fortunately, the Alan Guttmacher Institute, a private organization affiliated with the Planned Parenthood Federation, has been able to continue much of this work, as will be seen in other presentations in this book (see papers by Forrest, Henshaw).

ABORTION AND THE PUBLIC HEALTH

Abortion-related deaths had been declining in the United States since the 1950s, but the number of deaths decreased markedly after legalization in 1973 (Legge, 1985). There has been a continued decline of maternal deaths from all causes. This too is partially a benefit of legal abortion as women at high risk for pregnancy complications have been allowed to choose legal abortion. Paradoxically from the point of view of the anti-legal-abortion groups, legal abortion can be related to improvements in child health as well. In New York City it was possible to document a decrease in perinatal mortality, neonatal mortality, and infant mortality following legalization (Legge, 1985). The same trend to lower rates of infant deaths followed legalization in the U.S. as a whole, but is less easily attributed to legal abortion because of the introduction of social programs prior to 1973 which also improved child health.

FACTORS AFFECTING SAFETY OF ABORTION

Legal abortion is demonstrably safer than illegal abortion (CDC, 1979). Early abortion is safer than later abortion, i.e., the risk of complications and death increases with gestational age. Overall, the death rate from legal abortion performed in the first trimester of pregnancy has been only one material death per 100,000 abortions. Choice of procedure also influences risk. In the U.S. vacuum curettage has been preferred and it is safer than the older technique of sharp curettage. The experience of the surgeon is important. Perforation is more common when abortion is performed by trainees than by experienced surgeons (Grimes et al., 1984). Clearly the pattern of practice in the U.S. has for the most part favored abortion safety. The majority of abortions (90% by 1981) are performed in the first trimester, and the majority of these are performed in free-standing clinics by surgeons with great experience. A further safety factor is the use of local as opposed to general anesthesia. General anesthesia increases the risk of perforation, hemorrhage, major visceral injury, and death (Peterson et al., 1981).

An important innovation in technology was accomplished in the United States by Harvey Karman in the early 1970s. This was the development of the small, soft plastic cannula with a 50 cc plastic syringe as the vacuum source (Karman and Potts, 1972). This technique allowed safe, early abortion without dilatation and with minimal risk. Its use throughout the world is described in other papers of this symposium.

The technology for midtrimester abortion was initially inadequate. Practice in the early 1970s was to perform either hysterotomy, a major surgical procedure, or amnioinfusion of hypertonic saline for the midtrimester. Women presenting for abortion at 13–15 weeks were routinely delayed until 16 weeks or later since amnioinfusion was difficult prior to 16 weeks. This practice was documented in national statistics, which showed very few abortions performed in the 13–15-week range and then a substantial number performed at or after 16 weeks. The error of this practice was demonstrated by Tietze and Lewit in the first JPSA report (1972): curettage procedures performed at 13–14 weeks were only slightly riskier than the same procedure at 11–12 weeks, and much safer than saline infusion. In spite of the bias against curettage procedures in the midtrimester, several North American experts perfected the technique. Among them were Barr, Hanson, Hern, and Peterson (Stubblefield, 1981). By the late 1970s, the CDC could demonstrate the safety of these procedures over all others for midtrimester abortion (Grimes et al., 1977). As a result of the CDC scholarship and the teachings of a small number of practitioners skilled in midtrimester curettage, the procedure has become established. By 1981, Dilatation and Curettage (D&C) was the method of choice for abortions prior to 21 menstrual weeks (CDC, 1983). A variety of techniques are used for midtrimester D&C abortions. They differ primarily in whether or not the cervix is treated with laminaria tents or forcibly dilated (Stubblefield, 1981; Hern, 1984). In our institution, we have been able to teach a D&C technique to residents in training in obstetrics and gynecology. Under close faculty supervision a large number of midtrimester abortions has been performed with very few complications (Altman et al., 1985). The essentials of our technique are overnight treatment with laminaria tents, use of local anesthesia with low-dose intravenous sedation as opposed to general anesthesia, use of a large-bore vacuum cannula system, psychological preparation of the patient and good nursing support, and hands-on supervision by a small number of interested faculty.

SITE OF ABORTION AND SAFETY

First trimester abortions are performed more often in freestanding clinics or physicians' offices than in hospitals. Grimes and colleagues studied risk of death from abortion performed in the two settings. Overall the risk of death from first trimester abortion in a hospital was 1.5 per 100,000, while the risk was 0.6/100,000 for out-of-hospital abortions. Corrected for preexisting risk factors and concurrent surgery for tubal sterilization, the risk was the same in both locations (Grimes et al., 1981). Subsequent studies found that early midtrimester D&C procedures were as safely performed out of hospital as in, and the U.S. Supreme Court was convinced in 1983 to declare invalid those state laws which limited midtrimester abortion to the hospital setting.

The use of prophylactic antibiotics at the time of abortion appears to reduce the rate of infective complications. The rate of infection after abortion has been low in the U.S., but any postabortal infection could be serious and jeopardize later reproduction. Hodgson and colleagues demonstrated the efficacy of prophylactic tetracycline but other studies gave inconsistent results (Hodgson et al., 1975). More recently, a CDC study with a very large data set confirmed the benefit of the widespread practice of using prophylactic antibiotics (Schulz et al., 1984).

In our population, prevention of sensitization to the Rh blood group is an important consideration in providing abortion services. In U.S. abortion clinics, standard practice is to determine Rh blood group and to administer Rh immune globulin to all Rh-negative women immediately after the abortion.

MANAGEMENT OF COMPLICATIONS

With experience we have learned that certain practices add considerably to the safety of abortion. One of these practices is the fresh examination of the aborted tissue by the operating surgeon immediately after the procedure (Burnhill and Armstead, 1978). This practice prevents failed abortion and allows detection of patients at risk for ectopic pregnancy, a great concern in our setting.

We have also learned to treat the postabortal triad of pain, bleeding, and low-grade fever with prompt repeat curettage in the freestanding clinic. In most cases, reevacuation reveals either retained tissue or blood clot. While some of these patients might eventually respond to antibiotics and uterotonic agents without curettage, the prompt response with uterine evacuation reassures the patient and physician that the problem has been solved (Stubblefield, 1978).

With the large volume of abortions performed under good medical supervision, new problems were recognized. The postabortal syndrome was described in 1974. This condition is a type of uterine atony which produces severe pain after abortion if the uterus fails to contract and becomes distended with blood clot. The treatment is immediate reevacuation (Sands and Burnhill, 1974).

Another aid to management has been the introduction of laparoscopy. We have learned from experience that the best management of uterine perforation or unexplained bleeding is prompt hospitalization and diagnostic laparoscopy. In many cases this allows completion of the abortion without further injury and avoids the need for laparotomy (Laursen and Birnbaum, 1973). When an extensive perforation has occurred, we have learned to manage the patient with conservative surgery and repair, rather than with hysterectomy as initially practiced after legalization.

IMPACT OF LEGAL ABORTION ON LATER PREGNANCY

Worldwide, there is still controversy as to whether women who have obtained abortions will be able to bear children normally thereafter. In the U.S. the consistent finding of large, well-controlled studies has been that there is no measurable increase in late reproductive sequelae (Hogue et al., 1982). Neither is there a measurable increase in infertility after abortion when postabortal women are compared to control groups (Stubblefield et al., 1984). The experience of Eastern Europe in years past suggested that sterility, prematurity, low birth weight, and ectopic pregnancy were frequent late complications of abortion. The myth of later complications dies hard, probably because there is an element of truth to it. If abortions are performed badly, with excessive dilatation and uterine injury, there may well be late sequelae.

From the point of view of women's health, the experience with legalized abortion in the United States has been very favorable. We have all but abolished death from abortion. Advances in technique and the development of good services for early abortion have allowed provision of this essential service to the majority of women in need of it. The fact that risk of death or complications from abortion remains greater for black women than white is evidence that there remain unserved populations in our country (CDC, 1983). Unfortunately, the controversy has increased over the years in spite of the obvious success of legal abortion as a health measure. Opposition by small groups often backed by wealth and power of the Catholic Church is fierce. Clinic violence has become a very serious problem; many clinics have been destroyed by arson and clinic workers are subject to threats. Abortion providers are withstanding these challenges through the support of their own organization, the National Abortion Federation. This area of our activity may also provide lessons for the rest of the world. We hope we will demonstrate how to preserve legal abortion once it has been obtained.

REFERENCES

Altman, A., Stubblefield, P. G., Schlam, J. F., et al. Midtrimester abortion with laminaria and vacuum evacuation on a teaching service. J. Reprod. Med. 30:601, 1985.

Burnhill, M. S., Armstead, J. W. Reducing the morbidity of vacuum aspiration abortion. Int. J. Gynecol. & Obstet. 16:204, 1978.

Grimes, D. A., Schulz, K. F., Cates, W. Jr., et al. Midtrimester abortion by dilatation and evacuation: A safe and practical alternative. Int. J. Gynecol. & Obstet. 296:1141, 1977.

Grimes, D. A., Cates, W. Jr., Selik, R. M. Abortion facilities and the risk of death. Fam. Plan. Perspectives 13:30, 1981.

Grimes, D. A., Shulz, K. F., Cates, W. Jr. Prevention of uterine perforation during curettage abortion. JAMA 251:2108, 1984.

Hern, W. M. Abortion Practice. J. B. Lippincott, Philadelphia, 1984.

Hodgson, J. E., Major, B., Portman, K., et al. Prophylactic use of tetracycline for first trimester abortion. Obstet. Gynecol. 45:574, 1975.

Hogue, C. J. R., Cates, W. Jr., Tietze, C. The effects of induced abortion on subsequent reproduction. Epid. Review 4:66, 1982.

Karman, H., Potts, M. Very early abortion using the syringe as vacuum source. Lancet 1:7759, 1972.

Lauersen, N. H., Birnbaum, S. Laparoscopy as a diagnostic and therapeutic technique in uterine perforation during first trimester abortion. Amer. J. Obstet. Gynec. 117:522, 1973.

Legge, J. S. Abortion Policy: An Evaluation of the Consequences for Maternal and Infant Health. State University of New York Press, Albany, 1985.

Peterson, H. B., Grimes, D. A., Cates, W. Jr., et al. Comparative risk of death from induced abortion at 12 weeks or less gestation performed with local versus general anesthesia. Amer. J. Obstet. Gynecol. 141:763, 1981.

Roe v. Wade, 410 U.S. 113, 1973.

Sands, R. X., Burnhill, M. S., Hakin-Elahin, F. Postabortal uterine atony. Obstet. Gynecol. 43:595, 1974.

Shulz, K. F., Grimes, D. A., Park, T., et al. Prophylactic antibiotics to prevent febrile complications of curettage abortion. Paper presented at the 8th annual meeting of the National Abortion Federation, Los Angeles, California, May 15th, 1984.

Stubblefield, P. G. Current technology for abortion. Curr. Prob. Obstet. Gynecol. 2:1, 1978.

Stubblefield, P. G. Midtrimester abortion for curettage procedures: An overview. In J. E. Hodgson, ed., Abortion and Sterilization: Medical and Social Aspects, p. 277, Academic Press, London, Grune and Stratton, New York, 1981.

Stubblefield, P. G., Monson, R. R., Schoenbaum, S. C., et al. Fertility after induced abortion: A prospective follow-up study. Obstet. Gynecol. 63:186, 1984.

Tietze, C., Lewit, S. Joint program for the study of abortion (JPSA): Early medical complications for legal abortion. Stud. Fam. Plan. 3:96, 1972.

EVOLUTION OF SECOND TRIMESTER ABORTION TECHNIQUES

Warren M. Hern

Director
Boulder Abortion Clinic
1130 Alpine
Boulder, Colorado 80302, U.S.A.

Second trimester abortion techniques have varied during the past century, but current practices are essentially refinements of methods practiced for decades. Anecdotal accounts from both Europe and the United States indicate that 19th century and early 20th century physicians employed surgical evacuation of the uterus by various instruments; laminaria was used in the 19th century but abandoned due to the risks of infection.

The use of intraamniotic saline was introduced in 1934 by Aburel and reintroduced by Csapo in 1966 in the United States. Shortly after, various other substances were introduced for intra-amniotic use: hyperosmolar glucose solution, urea, and prostaglandins. Satisfactory methods of sterilizing laminaria resulted in a reintroduction of that material.

In the early 1970s, various physicians including Bierer and Steiner, Sloame, Davis, Sopher, and Finks began performing dilatation and evacuation (D&E) abortions, sometimes using serial multiple laminaria treatment of the cervix; this method was used by Japanese physicians with considerable success. The history of these efforts has been described by Stubblefield (1981) and Hern (1984) elsewhere and will not be reviewed in detail.

Dependence on the intraamniotic infusion of hypertonic or hyperosmolar agents and/or prostaglandins has been replaced in the United States by the extensive use of D&E abortion, especially up to 20 menstrual weeks' gestation, and it is now routine for D&E abortion to be performed through 24 menstrual weeks gestation.

While there are a variety of methods and results, I will present here a method or combination of methods which I have used successfully for ten years for second trimester abortion.

SERIAL MULTIPLE LAMINARIA METHOD IN D&E ABORTION

In second trimester abortion, as in other surgical procedures, there are certain surgical principles that must be observed in order to prevent complications:

* Accurate preoperative diagnosis and evaluation

* A high level of operator skill

* Sound sterile technique

* Atraumatic surgical technique

* Thorough removal of devitalized tissue

* Careful postoperative supervision and follow-up

Most of these principles are obvious and self-explanatory. In the case of D&E abortion, the first principle indicates the routine use of ultrasound for preoperative diagnosis of fetal age. The third and fourth principles indicate the use of serial multiple laminaria technique prior to uterine evacuation in order to prevent trauma to the uterine cervix and to help assure complete evacuation of tissue from the uterus. Figure 1 shows a cervix widely dilated by the use of laminaria.

Patient support means individual or small group counseling with close counselor and nurse support during the procedure and recovery phases.

Preoperative ultrasound is essential to accurate preoperative evaluation. Preoperative evaluation includes accurate diagnosis of fetal age, fetal presentation, placental location, and the presence of any abnormalities such as hydatidiform mole or anencephaly.

Serial multiple laminaria treatment over 24 hours or two days prior to the procedure is extremely valuable in the prevention of complications such as cervical laceration, uterine perforation, and incomplete abortion. Postoperative evaluation of tissue to determine actual fetal age and completeness of the abortion is essential.

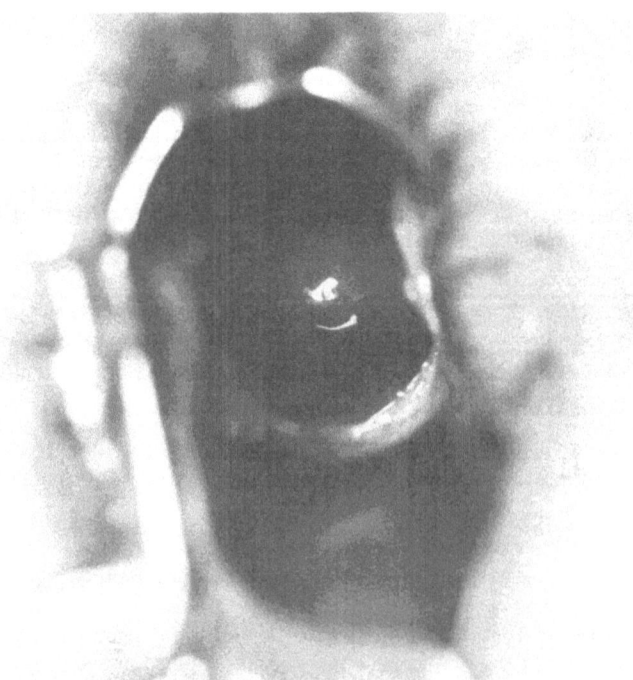

Fig. 1. Note lower lip of effaced cervix showing at bottom of bulging membranes.

From 20+ menstrual weeks on, I employ an intraamniotic infusion of 120 grams of hyperosmolar urea solution several hours prior to the D&E procedure.

Various instruments are used for this procedure. (Figs. 2—4)

Figure 5 shows the proper placement of multiple laminaria in the cervix. Figure 6 shows the result of placement of too many laminaria.

RESULTS

While we have performed more than 2,500 D&E procedures from 13 through 25 menstrual weeks' gestation, the results from 1000 patients from 17 through 25

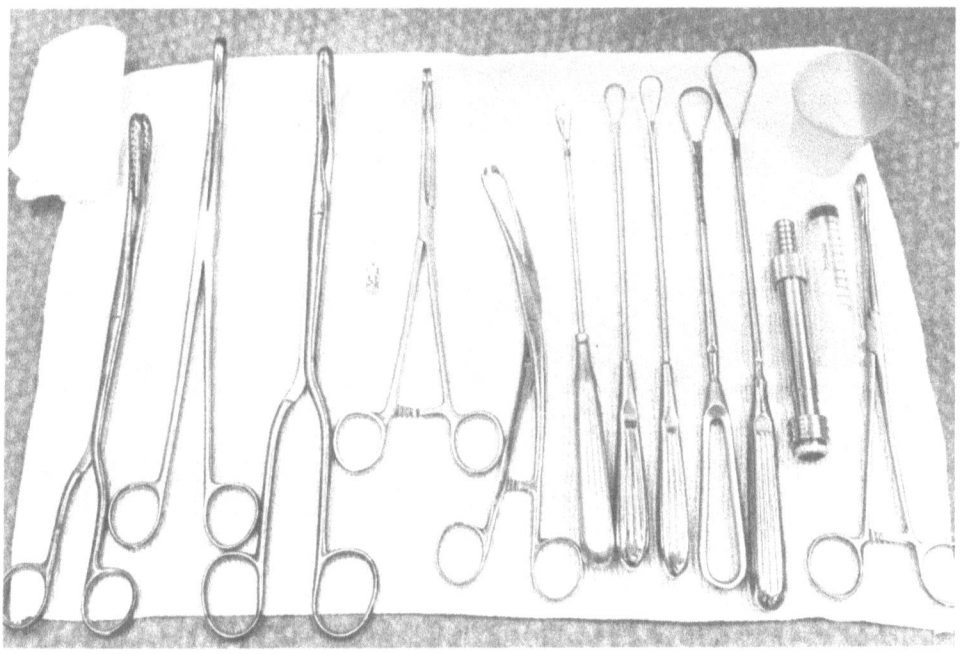

Fig. 2.

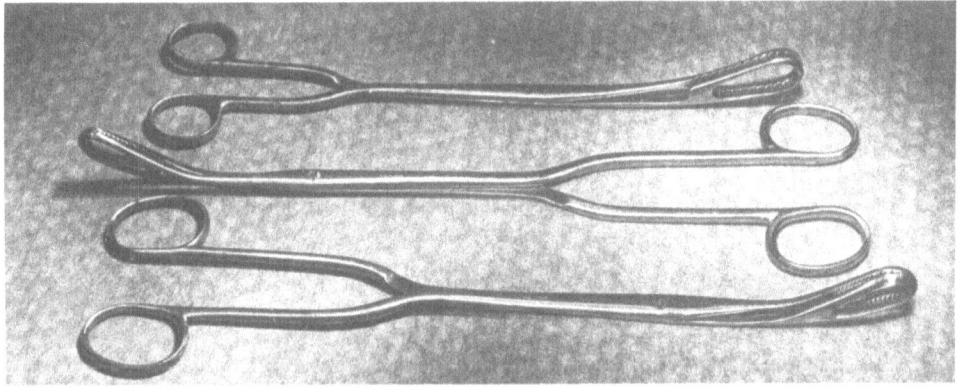

Fig. 3.

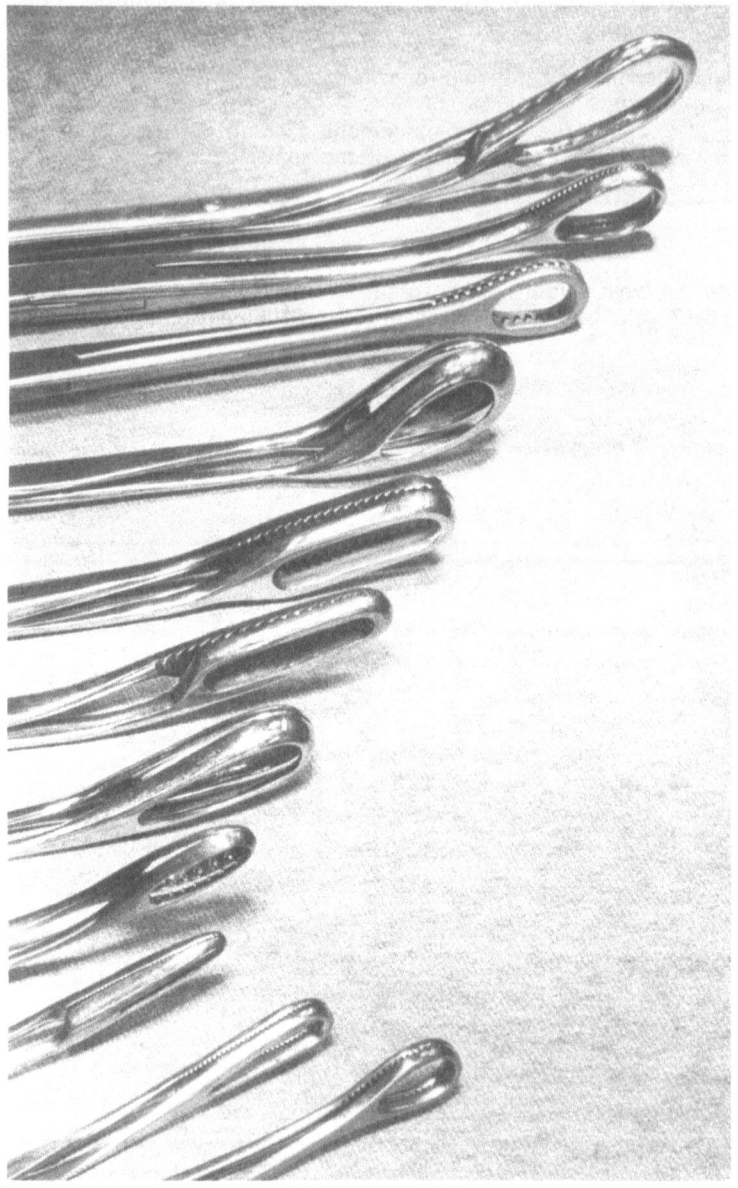

Fig. 4. Second-trimester D&E instrument table. From left:
Bierer, Kelley, large Hern, Foerster (Miltex), side curve
Kelly (Sklar), Sims Nos. 4–6 curettes, Bumm #4, Hunter
curette, Berkeley suction handle, straight Foerster forceps.

menstrual weeks, a range that includes the most difficult cases, gives a sense of
the results from this combination of methods (Hern, 1984a).

The final estimate of gestational age as defined by fetal foot length (Hern,
1984b) ranged from 17 through 25 menstrual weeks; 48.3 percent of the pregnancies
were from 17 through 19 menstrual weeks, and 50.6 percent were from 20 through
24 menstrual weeks. Twenty (2 percent) exceeded the intended gestational limit of
24 menstrual weks by one week due to errors in the preoperative diagnosis.

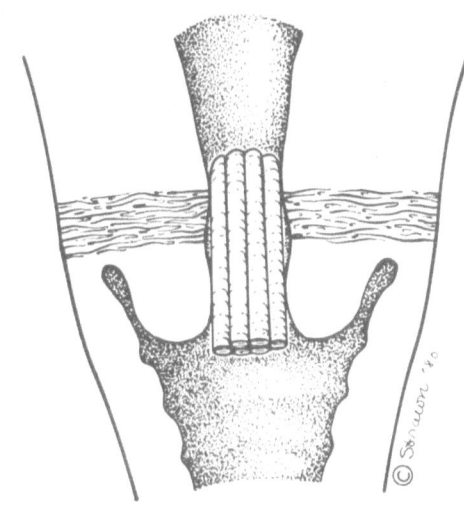

Fig. 5.

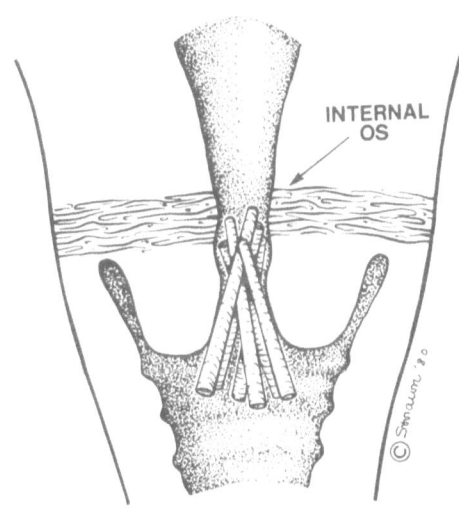

INTERNAL OS

Fig. 6.

Median dilatation and evacuation procedure time for all cases was 7.9 minutes, and medial blood loss was 149 ml with a mean of 172 ml. Procedure times were longer with pregnancies of more than 22 weeks' gestation, but blood loss was not increased (Table 1). Fetal weight ranged from 74 to 906 g, fetal foot length ranged from 23 to 49 mm, and biparietal diameter ranged from 32 to 63 mm.

Among patients receiving urea amnioinfusion, injection to procedure time ranged from 5.4 to 5.7 hours (Table 2), although some patients went into labour quickly and aborted within one or two hours after injection. There were no births of living fetuses.

Table 1: Procedure Characteristics (All Patients)

Gestational Age (wk from LMP)	No. of Patients (N = 1,000)	Median Procedure Time (min)	Median Blood loss (mL)
17	117	7.5	102
18	178	7.0	102
19	181	7.4	150
20	91	8.0	154
21	137	7.8	151
22	153	8.4	150
23	70	9.7	102
24	53	10.2	100
25	20	15.5	109
Total	1,000		

LMP = last menstrual period.

Table 2: Intra-amniotic Urea Infusion Followed by Dilatation and Evacuation

Gestational Age (wk from LMP	No. of Patients (N = 415)	Median Amniotic Fluid Withdrawn (mL)	Median Urea Injected (g)	Median Injection to Procedure Time (h)
20	40	280	104	5.4
21	96	227	83	5.3
22	142	300	118	5.4
23	64	327	118	5.2
24	53	378	120	5.5
25	20	328	119	5.7
Total	415			

LMP = last menstrual period.

Table 3: Overall Complication Rates*

Major complications** (N = 3)		0.3%
Minor complications (N = 55)		5.5%
Clinically identifiable infections (N = 6)		0.6%
Unsuspected retained tissue requiring treatment (N = 7)		0.7%
Reaspiration within 1 wk (N = 3)	0.3%	
Reaspiration beyond 1 wk (N = 4)	0.4%	
Reaspiration within 6 hrs, retained tissue (N = 20)		2.0%
Total blood loss of more than 500 mL (N = 18)		1.8%
1000+ mL (not including minor complications) (N = 2)	0.2%	
Cervical lacerations (N = 3)		0.3%
Coagulopathy (N = 1)		0.1%

* N = 1,000.
** Major complication = major unintended surgery, hemorrhage requiring transfusion, pelvic infection with two or more days of fever and a peak of at least 40°C or with hospitalization of 11 or more days.

Only three out of 1000 patients experienced a major complication for a major complication rate of 0.3 percent (Table 3). We are not aware of a lower reported major complication rate for late second trimester abortion in the medical literature.

CONCLUSION

There are no completely satisfactory methods of second trimester abortion. However, it is possible to obtain extremely low complication rates in second trimester abortion by the observation of important surgical principles. Application of these principles in second trimester D&E abortion includes the use of routine preoperative ultrasound, serial mutliple laminaria treatment of the cervix prior to abortion, and adjunctive urea amnioinfusion in late second trimester abortion.

REFERENCES

Stubblefield, P. G. Midtrimester abortion by curettage procedures: An overview. In Hodgson, J. E., ed., Abortion and Sterilization: Medical and Social Aspects, p. 277. Academic Press, London, 1981.

Hern, W. M. Abortion Practice. J. B. Lippincott Co., Philadelphia, 1984.

Hern, W. M. Serial multiple laminaria and adjunctive urea in late outpatient dilatation and evacuation abortion. Obstet. Gynecol. 63:543, 1984.

Hern, W. M. Correlation of fetal age and measurements between 10 and 26 weeks of gestation. Obstet. Gynecol. 63:26, 1984.

TRAINING PHYSICIANS IN ELECTIVE ABORTION

TECHNIQUE IN THE UNITED STATES

Philip D. Darney

Associate Professor of Obstetrics, Gynecology, and
    Reproductive Sciences
University of California, San Francisco
Medical Director, Family Planning Clinic
San Francisco General Hospital
San Francisco, California, U.S.A.

INTRODUCTION

The typical path for the dissemination of a new surgical technique is that an innovator (often an academic with time and funds for clinical research) develops a new technique, describes it at medical meetings and in the professional literature, and then teaches it to colleagues and surgeons-in-training. These students of the surgical innovator then teach it to their own students and the technique becomes incorporated into standard medical practice. Safe and effective techniques thus become generally recognized and accepted and are taught to successive generations of surgical trainees.

The history of training in abortion technique is, however, very different. Because abortion was illegal throughout the growth and development of modern institutions of medical education in the United States, it was never incorporated into the experience of students or post graduate trainees. Many gynecologists and generalists of this period were skilled illegal abortionists, but academic physicians, who are the writers of textbooks and teachers of new surgeons, were rarely familiar with abortion techniques.

Tietze estimated that about one half million illegal abortions were performed yearly in the United States prior to legalization. Complication rates from these illegal abortions were high, but not high enough to suggest that all abortionists were incompetent by today's standards. However, when abortion became legal, the skilled abortionists were not in medical schools where they might have been able to provide training to new surgeons. Nor did academic departments of obstetrics and gynecology welcome skilled abortionists to their ranks. Even though abortion was now legal, a stigma remained on those who had earlier performed illegal abortions. Training programs for new obstetrician-gynecologists did not incorporate abortion training into their teaching. Abortion was sometimes considered a simple procedure no different from standard dilatation and curettage performed for diagnostic purposes. In 1973, Burkman et al. observed "it appears that a significant number of residents are not exposed to the management of elective abortions." The writers drew this conclusion after surveying 86 university departments of obstetrics and gynecology. Teaching hospitals were surveyed again in 1976 by Lindheim and Cotterill. They sent questionnaires to the directors of all 438 hospital-based residency programs in the United States. Only half responded, but they appeared representa-

tive of all such hospitals. The authors concluded that "even the maximum estimates show that a substantial minority of residents are not being trained to perform abortions, while the lowest estimate suggests that more than 4 in 10 residents
may not." A third survey (Darney, et al., 1986) to which 86 percent of U.S. teaching hospitals responded in 1985 showed improvement, but still nearly one-third of
the programs answered that they did not provide training in abortion.

A problem for hospitals that do provide training in abortion procedures is
often that their number of abortions is too small to accomplish adequate training.
In 1973 Burkman estimated that "less than 8 percent" of the elective abortions
estimated for the United States were performed in the university hospitals surveyed. A more recent analysis by Henshaw, et al. (1984), reported that in 1982
only 18 percent of all U.S. abortions took place in hospital facilities. As Burkman,
et al. (1973), point out, the numbers of abortions performed in most teaching hospitals are so small that adequate training may be difficult to provide even if the
faculty is interested in doing so. The conclusion reached by several authors (Burkman, et al., 1973; Lindheim, Cotterill, 1978; Henshaw, et al., 1984) is that hospitals
have lagged behind free standing clinics as both providers and teachers of abortion
technique.

This situation is the converse of that which usually introduces advances in
medical care: academics in hospitals develop new techniques which are disseminated to non-hospital-based clinicians. Why was the situation different with regard
to abortion? As mentioned earlier, illegal abortion had, of course, not been a
hospital-based procedure. When abortion was legalized hospitals were slow to meet
the demand for this new service, while free-standing clinics were rapidly established in most major cities throughout the U.S.A. As Nathanson and Becker (1980)
point out, "abortion as a legitimate hospital service can be conceived as an innovation." These authors found that when gynecologists themselves did not promote
abortion services in a hospital, the perceived social risk attached to the performance of abortions was sufficient to prevent them from being offered or to insure
that few were performed. A few teaching hospitals did establish abortion services,
but most did not. The academic physicians responsible for the services provided in
medical school-affiliated hospitals were usually not themselves familiar with abortion techniques, and were extremely unlikely to invite the abortionists who were
familiar with them to teach the techniques. Consequently, abortion services and
the training of physicians--mostly private practitioners and moonlighting resi-
dents--took place in free standing abortion clinics that had no affiliation with
residency training programs. Soon these clinics were providing a million abortions
yearly in the United States. Their techniques, experiences, and complication rates
were well documented in the medical literature (e.g., Hodgson, 1975; Nathanson,
1972; Walton, 1972; Wulff and Freiman, 1977), but none of these accounts described
hospital-based abortion services.

The assertion that abortion was too simple a procedure to warrant formal
training was not supported by the facts. Complication rates were significantly
higher when resident physicians performed abortions (Schultz, Grimes, Cates, 1983;
Grimes, Schultz, Cates, 1984). As abortion procedures developed to allow second
trimester uterine evacuations, the need for training became even more obvious
(Cates, Schultz, Grimes, et al., 1972), but few resident physicians received formal
training in abortion.

As time passed after the legalization of abortion in the U.S.A., the abortion
clinics were recognized as providing an efficient and safe service. More and more
public and private insurers reimbursed them, and the clinics were busy and prosper-
ing. A few teaching hospitals perceived the need for abortion services and recognized that funding was available. Some of these hospitals began to perform abortions, usually in operating rooms where costs were high and staff attitudes toward
abortion often negative. Resident physicians were sometimes given the task of
performing these abortions, but were poorly supervised because the academic physicians were not themselves sufficiently skilled in this procedure. In some teaching

departments, the attending physicians learned abortion techniques and organized clinics but did not include residents because teaching abortion had no academic stature and made the clinic less efficient.

This latter situation prevailed in the teaching program described below. The great majority of abortions were performed by attending physicians who had low complication rates. Occasionally, when attending physicians were unavailable, resident physicians performed first trimester abortions, but when they did so their complication rates were considerably higher than those of the attending physicians (2.2 vs. 7.4 percent). This discovery prompted organization of a training program for the resident staff initially in early abortion and subsequently in second trimester abortion. The training techniques and the results of the program are described below.

CHARACTERISTICS OF THE TRAINING PROGRAM

Two questions which must be answered at the outset are "Who should be trained?" and "Who should do the training?" In a typical four year obstetrics and gynecology residency training program, first year residents learn the rudiments of medical and surgical care. Second post graduate year trainees may not have sufficient surgical skill to operate rapidly under local anesthesia; fourth year residents are likely to be involved in more complicated surgical cases and administration of junior residents. Third year residents, therefore, seem ideal for receiving training in the abortion clinic.

Since the unit had been functioning for four years with attending physicians performing abortions, these physicians were logical choices to train the residents. Experience in other residency training programs (Altman, et al., 1985) has demonstrated that abortion training is best accomplished when "a small but experienced faculty group" provides "direct, hands-on supervision" of resident physicians. These statements may seem obvious, but some hospital abortion programs rely on faculty who are not themselves sufficiently experienced and do not have a high level of interest in abortion care.

The hospital operating room model is not conducive to providing abortion services or teaching abortion technique. Operating rooms are expensive and inefficient for procedures of short duration, and they are frightening to patients having operations under local anesthesia. A much more efficient and acceptable model is that of the free standing abortion clinic as described by Landy and Lewitt (1982). In order for hospital-based post graduate trainees to learn modern methods of elective abortion, it is necessary to establish an out-patient-like setting within the hospital. The training program described here had inaugurated an out-patient abortion service based on the free standing clinic model prior to initiating the training of residents. Other training programs (Altman et al., 1985) had established such clinics after discovering that resident training in abortion was unsatisfactory in the operating room setting.

The abortion clinic model generally includes counseling, nursing, and physician staff (Bruce, 1981; Landy, Lewitt, 1982). Counselors provide informed consent and emotional support and serve as patient advocates. Nurses organize and maintain equipment and medication supplies, administer pre- and post-operative medications, assist the surgeon, and monitor post-operative recovery. Physicians, usually gynecologists, perform pre-operative assessments, carry out the abortion, and provide treatment and follow-up of complicated cases. Local anesthesia is often employed because of greater safety, although general anesthesia can also be used in this setting. Patients spend only a few hours at the clinic and receive prolonged observation only when complications occur. Almost all clinics use suction evacuation abortion in the first trimester. Those performing later abortions almost always use the cervical dilatation and instrumental uterine evacuation abortion technique (D and E).

The training program described here uses protocols following these general guidelines. Since post graduate trainees are expected to learn first and second trimester abortion techniques in a period of six weeks, they are guided by experienced faculty and standardized protocols governing equipment and medications. Many variations are possible, but the equipment and medications schedule shown in Table 1 are typical and function well in the training situation described here.

Women seeking pregnancy termination discuss the risks of and alternatives to abortion and learn about the abortion procedure from an experienced counselor. If they choose to go ahead with the abortion, they sign a consent form for either first or second trimester abortion which specifically outlines the risks and possible complications of each procedure. Since all patients receive pre-operative cervical dilation with hydrophilic dilators (laminaria tents or hypan dilators), they undergo a physical examination and dilator insertion by the resident or the attending physician prior to the abortion. Patients thus meet, before the operation, both the counselor who will provide emotional support and the physician who will perform the abortion.

Table 1: Instruments, Equipment, Supplies, and
Medications for Abortion Procedures

Instruments recommended for each first trimester tray:

Graves medium open-sided vaginal speculum
Bierer atraumatic tenaculum
Foerster sponge forcep--curved
Pratt or Denniston cervical dilators, sizes 13 through 43 French
medicine bowl (50 ml) for local anesthetic
stainless steel bowl (500 ml) for cleansing solution
uterine curette, Sims, size 2

Equipment which should be immediately available but not present on every tray:

vaginal retractors, Heaney, medium size
needle holder, Heaney, long
tissue forcep, long
Sopher forcep, large serrations
uterine sound
uterine curette, Sims, sizes 3 & 4

Disposable equipment and supplies recommended for each procedure:

chloroprocaine (Nesacaine, 1%) 15 ml
fentanyl, 0.1 mg (2 ml) or butorphanol 2 mg (1 ml)
atropine, 0.4 mg (1 cc)
syringe, plastic (10 cc) with control grip for paracervical block
syringe, 5 cc, for intravenous administration of analgesics
needle, 25 g (1-1/2") for paracervical block
needle, 25 g (1/2") for intravenous medications
gauze sponges, 4"x4" (5)
cotton balls (5)
clear plastic collection tubing with clear plastic handle, 11 mm inside diameter
cannulas, uterine evacuation, rigid, clear plastic, 8 mm through 12 mm outside diameter, straight and curved
cannulas, whistle-tip, flexible plastic, 5 mm through 8 mm outside diameter

At the time of the operation the patient may choose to have a partner, friend, or relative present. Sometimes a medical student may observe with the patient's consent. The clinic staff (counselor, nurse, and physician) maintain a tranquil environment in the operating room: extraneous noise and conversation is kept to a minimum, the room is dimly illuminated except where bright lights focus on the operating field, music which promotes relaxation is played, the counselor sits at the head of the table to comfort and inform the patient. The nurse administers intravenous fentanyl (0.1 milligrams) and atropine (0.4 milligrams) directly intravenously through a 25 gauge needle. Intravenous infusions are initiated rarely as required for administration of antibiotics or uterotonic agents, or to treat dehydration or blood loss.

Trainees are taught to perform operations rapidly so that patients do not have prolonged discomfort. Counselors time each procedure and inform the physician of the elapsed time between onset of suction evacuation and final removal of the speculum. The administration of the paracervical block is not included in timing the operation because trainees should not be encouraged to undertake the operation before the block has achieved satisfactory analgesia (at least 2 minutes with chloroprocaine 1 percent, 10 milliliters). At the conclusion of the abortion, the physician is responsible for removing the specimen container from the aspiration machine and taking it and all equipment to the adjacent "dirty" equipment room. There the physician examines the specimen, taking care to determine that the patient is no longer pregnant and that the abortion is complete. Whenever possible, the length of the fetal foot is measured and correlated with duration of gestation so that trainees can judge their success in accurately assessing gestational age prior to the abortion. The physician also places the specimen in a container for pathological examination and places dirty instruments in receptacles. Nursing and counseling staff are not burdened with disposing of tissue and dirty instruments, but devote their entire attention to the support of patients.

Trainees initially observe both first and second trimester abortions performed by the attending physician. The attending physician then observes and instructs the trainee in several first trimester abortions. Later on, the trainee accomplishes these abortions alone but the attending physician is immediately available for advice and consultation. Second trimester abortions require a more complicated technique and special instruments for uterine evacuation. They also have a higher rate of serious complications. Therefore, trainees never perform these abortions without direct supervision, and they gradually acquire experience with early gestations before progressing to terminations later in gestation. A satisfactory approach is to have trainees begin at 14 or 15 weeks and advance no more than two weeks in gestation with each subsequent procedure. Direct sonographic guidance of intrauterine instruments is employed for all second trimester uterine evacuations. Operations are not begun unless the attending physician agrees that cervical dilation is adequate for a safe and rapid procedure. If complications necessitate re-evacuation or laparotomy, the attending physician and the trainee undertake these procedures together, so that the trainee acquires experience with the causes and treatment of complications. At the end of the six week training period, the trainee will have performed approximately 100 first trimester abortions and 25 second trimester abortions from 15 through 22 menstrual weeks gestation.

RESULTS OF THE ABORTION TRAINING PROGRAM

Prior to the initiation of the training program, resident physicians performing unsupervised first trimester abortions had complication rates higher than those reported in large series (Hodgson, 1975; Wulff, Freiman, 1977). Table 2 shows first and second trimester abortion complication rates for all surgeons including residents during 1979-80 and 1983-84, before and after institution of the teaching program. Complications were defined as occurrence of uterine perforation, the need for uterine re-evacuation or the need to hospitalize the patient. After initiating the training program, complication rates for residents declined dramatically and complication rates for attending surgeons declined modestly.

Table 2: First and Second Trimester Abortion Complication* Rates (%) and
Number of Abortions (N) by Surgeon before (1979-80) and after (1983-84)
Initiation of Teaching Program

Surgeon	Before (1979-80)		After (1983-84)	
	%	N	%	N
Residents	7.4	75	0.7	979
A	2.9	559	1.7	229
B	3.4	377	--	--
C	0.4	225	--	--
D	--	--	1.6	433
E	--	--	1.7	190
F	--	--	1.4	138
All Surgeons	2.7	1,236	1.7	1,969

* Perforation, reevacuation, or hospitalization.
-- Did not do abortions during this period.

Table 3 examines complication rates for second trimester abortions before and during the teaching program. Prior to the teaching program, all second trimester abortions were performed by experienced attending gynecologists. After the teaching program, most, but not all second trimester abortions were performed by resident physicians under direct supervision of an attending physician and with the use of intraoperative sonography. Complication rates for perforation, transfusion, and infection declined, but the rate of uterine re-evacuation increased. The rate of laparotomies required for serious complications at the time of second trimester abortion also declined (see Table 4) from 8.6 percent prior to the program to 2.2 percent during the teaching program.

DISCUSSION

There are explanations other than the teaching program for the decline in rates of complications from 1979-80 to 1983-84. Table 3 shows that the complication rates for both attending physicians and for resident trainees decreased over this period, but not nearly as much as did the rate for the residents. This secular trend suggests that at least a portion of the decline in complication rates was due to factors other than improved resident training. It is possible that the attending physicians who were active in the teaching program became more competent than those who had not participated in it. An explanation for the somewhat surprising finding that resident trainees' complication rates were lower than those for attending physicians is that attending physicians were likely to perform or intervene in a higher proportion of complicated first and second trimester abortions. It seems quite likely that the routine use of intraoperative sonography for later second trimester abortions not only helped the teaching program but also reduced the rate of serious complications for resident and attending physicians alike. The only complication which increased in incidence after the institution of the training program was uterine re-evacuation. This finding is probably due to a more aggressive program of uterine re-evacuation in the clinic in order to avoid subsequent hospital admission, the rates for which declined after the training program began.

CONCLUSION

Examination of rates for several types of complications occurring in a teaching hospital-based abortion clinic show that rates were signicantly lower for resi-

Table 3: Second Trimester Abortion Complications and Rates (%) and
Number of Cases (N) before (1979-80) and after (1983-84)
Initiation of Teaching Program

Complications	1979-80		1983-84	
	%	N	%	N
Perforation	0.59	4	0.35	2
Transfusion	0.45	3	0.27	1
Infection	1.49	10	0.71	4
Reevacuation	0.74	5	1.96	11
Hospital Admission	1.78	12	1.25	7
Total 2nd Trimester Abortions	672		560	

Table 4: Second Trimester Abortions (16 to 23 Weeks) Requiring Exploratory
Laparotomies before (1979-80) and after (1983-84)
Initiation of Teaching Program

	1979-80	1983-84
Laparotomies	7	2
Abortions	810	889
Rate/1,000	8.6	2.2

dent physicians after training than before training. Although there are other possible explanations for the change, they seem unlikely to account for all of the improvement in resident performance. The findings demonstrate that first and second trimester abortion techniques can be improved by training and that, when properly supervised, trainees can accomplish these procedures safely.

The training program described here has several components which were important to its success: the trainers were experienced in doing abortions and believed that they had specific skills to impart to resident trainees. The trainees were senior residents who had already acquired dexterity with surgical instruments and who had had considerable experience performing routine curettage for diagnostic and therapeutic purposes under general anesthesia. The program was organized on a clinic model away from the operating room so that residents could learn techniques of local anesthesia and rapid uterine evacuation. The efficient use of their time allowed them to perform an adequate number of abortions in a short period. A support staff including counselors and nurses dedicated to efficient and compassionate care of abortion patients helped attending and resident physicians to provide care under the most favorable circumstances. Finally, standardized protocols insured that appropriate instruments, equipment, and medications were always employed. These six components were critical to the success of the training program.

ACKNOWLEDGMENTS

The author wishes to thank Ms. Susan Leary for reviewing patient records of 1979-80 and Ms. Blair Darney for reviewing those of 1983-84.

REFERENCES

Altman, A. M., Stubblefield, P. G., Schlam, J. F., et al. Midtrimester abortion with Laminaria and vacuum evacuation on a teaching service. J. Repro. Med. 30:601, 1985.

Bruce, J. Women-oriented health care. New Hampshire Feminist Health Center, Stud. Fam. Plan. 12:353, 1981.

Burkman, R. T., King, T. M., Burnett, L. S., et al. University abortion programs: One year later. Am. J. Obstet. Gynecol. 119:131, 1974.

Cates, W., Jr., Schulz, K. F., Grimes, D. A., et al. Dilatation and evacuation procedures and second trimester abortions. JAMA 248:559, 1982.

Darney, P. D., Landy, U., Lewit, S., Sweet, R. L. A survey of obstetrics and gynecology residency programs' elective abortion teaching practices. Manuscript in preparation, 1986.

Grimes, D. A., Schulz, K. F., Cates, W., Jr. Prevention of uterine perforation during curettage abortion. JAMA 251:2108, 1984.

Henshaw, S. K., Forrest, J. D., Blaine, E. Abortion services in the United States, 1981 and 1982. Fam. Plan. Persp. 16:119, 1984.

Hodgson, J. E. Major complications of 20,248 consecutive first trimester abortions: Problems of fragmented care. Adv. Plan. Parenthood 9:52, 1975.

Landy, U., Lewit, S. Administrative, counseling and medical practices in National Abortion Federation facilities. Fam. Plan. Persp. 14:257, 1982.

Lindheim, B. L., Cotterill, M. A. Training in induced abortion by obstetrics and gynecology residency programs. Fam. Plan. Persp. 10:24, 1978.

Nathanson, B. N. Ambulatory abortion: Experience with 26,000 cases (July 1, 1970 to August 1, 1971). N. Engl. J. Med. 286:403, 1972.

Nathanson, C., Becker, M. H. Obstetricians' attitudes and hospital abortion services. Fam. Plan. Persp. 12:26, 1980.

Schulz, K. F., Grimes, D. A., Cates, W., Jr. Measures to prevent cervical injury during suction curettage abortion. Lancet 1:1182, 1983.

Walton, L. A. Immediate morbidity on a large abortion service: The first year's experience. NYS J. Med. 72:919, 1972.

Wulff, G. J. L., Freiman, S. M. Elective abortion: Complications seen in a free-standing clinic. Obstet. Gynecol. 49:351, 1977.

REDUCING THE RISKS OF PREGNANCY TERMINATION

Michael S. Burnhill

Professor of Clinical Obstetrics and Gynecology
UMDNJ--Robert Wood Johnson Medical School
New Brunswick, New Jersey, U.S.A.

The intense interest that has been focused around legal abortion in the United States has had some extraordinarily beneficial side effects. Perhaps the most important has been the systematic scientific monitoring of abortion morbidity and mortality. Christopher Tietze (to whom this seminar and paper were dedicated) was the patron saint of abortion surveillance. The Joint Program for the Study of Abortion (JPSA) was the first to look at the medical consequences of legal abortion. His pioneering work was continued and expanded by the Abortion Surveillance Division of the Centers for Disease Control (Cates, Grimes, 1981a, 1981b; Grimes, Cates, 1979; Peterson et al., 1981). In addition to the national data, in-depth analysis was provided by comprehensive reviews of the performance of some of the larger not-for-profit freestanding abortion centers (Burnhill, 1978a).

The collecting of data was initially viewed with great expectations by advocates of abortion (who felt that the studies would show that abortion is reasonably safe) and foes of abortion (who expected that the burden of suddenly providing millions of abortions would result in a disastrously high rate of complications). To the surprise of both sides of the issue, abortion has proved to be an exceedingly safe operation.

After the initial excitement of developing de novo a new type of consumer-sensitive medical care delivery system other uses for the data became apparent. For literally the first time in history, it became possible to study performance and result outcomes for a surgical procedure. Complications--rates and types--were analyzed by age, parity, race, previous medical history, duration of gestation of the patient, type of procedure carried out, technique used, training and experience of the surgeon. Elsewhere in surgery, little interest had been evinced in detailed analysis of outcomes, partially because no large computerized data base had been collected, and partially because of the surgeons' reluctance to have their shortcomings and problems exposed to public scrutiny.

The availability of the data and the extraordinary interest shown by the public in serious abortion complications and deaths alerted thoughtful providers to the possibilities of still further reducing abortion complications by studying individual aspects of the abortion procedure and choosing those techniques that produced less trauma. The study of complications also resulted in the development of methods designed to minimize the medical, social, psychological, political, legal, and financial sequelae of any particular complication.

Beginning in 1979, the fledgling National Abortion Federation began to sponsor workshops designed to expose providers to the means of averting and managing complications. From these early workshops, the concept of "Risk Management" in abortion developed (Darney, 1984; Oliva, 1980; Soderstrom et al., 1984). Similar techniques were later used for training in family planning, sterilization, and other areas of medicine and surgery.

WHAT IS "RISK MANAGEMENT"?

It is the science and art of preventing complications and reducing their sequelae by careful prospective planning.

HOW IS IT USED IN PROVIDING ABORTION SERVICES?

Risk Management Principles are applied in the following areas of the provision of abortion services:

1. Facility design.

2. Choice of appropriate equipment.

3. Training and evaluation of providers.

4. Selection of patients.

5. Precise estimation of gestational age.

6. Use of safer techniques.

7. Monitoring of patients during and after procedure.

8. Inspection of products of conception.

9. Triage of high-risk patients and follow-up after procedure.

This brief overview will only survey those areas where risk management procedures are of use. Two somewhat larger examples will be given: the use of osmotic dilators for cervical dilation, and the examination of tissue immediately after the procedure. For more extended and in-depth coverage, the reader is referred to: Burnhill (1975; 1978a, 1978b, 1979a, 1979b, 1986), Hern (1981), Hodgson (1981), LaFerla (1986), McIntosh (1984), Stubblefield (1979), and Zatuchni et al. (1979).

To apply risk management principles, one must face the inevitability of problems and complications. Preparation involves planning, supplying, rehearsing, and evaluating. This, in turn, mandates expending time, money, and effort. What is most needed, however, is commitment to provide quality and excellence of care. Of course, there is a payoff for all this effort: better results imply fewer problems, better morale, lower medical costs, healthier patients, and, last but not least, less litigation. Let me then review the areas that need attention if one is to safely perform abortions.

Faulty Design

While many things can be said about the use of color, flow patterns, space, etc., two overriding design requirements exist:

1. To be able to rapidly transfer a patient to an ambulance for emergency care.

2. To be able to safely evacuate the facility in the event of fire or other catastrophic phenomenon.

Choosing Appropriate Equipment

Reliable state-of-the-art medical and laboratory equipment--especially those needed for emergencies--drugs, intravenous supplies, airways, etc., must be stocked. Fresh (unexpired) medication--whose location is known and accessible to personnel trained in their use--is vital.

Training and Evaluation of Providers

As a general rule, physicians, including gynecologists, are ill prepared to safely perform abortions. This means that formal training is generally required before evacuation procedures can be safely performed (Hern, 1981). Further training is required if more advanced procedures are performed (Burnhill, 1978b; Grimes et al., 1984; Hern, 1981). Additionally, the complication rate for each physician should be calculated and compared to others in the clinic or to national averages. Some physicians do not have the skill or personality to properly perform an abortion, others may have sudden or gradual deterioration in their competency if exposed to personal stress or psychologic deterioration.

Selection of Patients

It goes without saying (but I will anyway) that the woman must want an abortion and will have made the choice knowingly and by her own free will (having been aware of the alternatives).

She must be physically and mentally well enough to have the procedure performed in a freestanding facility.

Some patients need special attention and some abortions should only be performed in a hospital.

Examples of high and higher risk patients include: addicts, alcoholics, psychotics, the chronically and severely ill, and febrile patients. Other high-risk conditions are: morbid obesity, active asthma, poorly controlled diabetes or epilepsy, cardiac arrhythmia, and pelvic inflammatory disease.

Estimation of Gestational Age

One of the best documented relationships is that of increasing gestational age and the rate of complications (Burnhill et al., 1978a; Cates and Grimes, 1981a; Grimes and Cates, 1979). The last menstrual period date is frequently erroneous due to a patient's memory gaps, lying, or bleeding after conception. Pelvic exam estimates are distorted by obesity, retroversion of the uterus, abdominal wall rigidity, myomas, cysts, hydramnios, multiple gestation, and hydatid mole.

The development of extremely reliable monoclonal antibody based pregnancy tests has more or less eliminated procedures performed on nonpregnant patients and has somewhat simplified the identification of ectopic pregnancy.

Ultrasonic examination is the ultimate unraveller of gestational mystery. I cannot recommend strongly enough the use of ultrasonic evaluation--there is no reasonable or prudent substitute for this technique. Unless the service is limited to early termination (i.e., less than 10−12 weeks), it would generally pay for any reasonably busy clinic (even in poorer countries) to be sure that diagnostic ultrasound is available.

Use of Safer Technique

Abortion techniques are reviewed in the previously mentioned general references on abortion. In addition, I would like to briefly discuss the use of osmotic dilators. The experienced clinician has long appreciated the dilatation produced by using laminaria sticks. They are of inestimable value for hypoplastic or stenotic cervices or when wide cervical dilation is needed as in advanced dilation and evacuation (D&E).

Schultz et al. (1983) and Grimes et al. (1984) demonstrated on a scientific basis that the risks of upper genital tract injury was reduced about 75 percent when laminaria was used.

Though still very useful, the laminaria produced from the North Sea (Digitatum) and the Japan Sea (Japonicum) are slow acting and not clearly predictable in their swelling time. Lamicell[R], a magnesium sulfate impregnated plastic foam, produces cervical softening but has not achieved wide acceptance. Most recently, Dilapan[R] has been marketed. This is a hygroscopic dilator based on an osmotic hypan plastic material. Burnhill and Robinson (1984) and Burnhill and Danon (1985) showed that the dilator swells more readily and to a greater amount than the natural vegetation. The author feels that plastic of this type will be the material of choice when an osmotic dilator is needed or required.

Patient Monitoring

It seems redundant to remind providers that patients need to be monitored during and after procedures. However, occasionally, because of the staff's or physician's fatigue, stress, or boredom, the condition of an individual woman may pass unobserved or disregarded. Amongst the warning signs are tachycardia; bradycardia; cardiac irregularities; hyperventilation; apnea; weak pulse; decreased blood pressure; alterations in consciousness such as drowsiness, loss of consciousness, syncope, seizures, loss of orientation, fuzzy or bizarre responses; extreme agitation; increased, abnormal, or peculiarly located pain; nausea or vomiting; coldness of extremities; sweating.

Any one or more of these signs and symptoms may only be a manifestation of increased anxiety, but their very presence mandates increased and more careful observation. One may be able to avert cardiopulmonary failure, cardiac arrest, brain damage from anaphylactic reaction secondary to the use of local anesthesia, increased visceral damage from uterine perforation, or hemorrhagic shock.

This article will not go into any further detail into the prevention and management of these life-threatening complications. The points are:

1. Alterations in a patient's general condition need to be observed, monitored, recorded, and managed.

2. Equipment for supporting the circulation, maintaining oxygenation, treating anaphylaxis, etc., needs to be immediately available and in good working condition.

3. Personnel trained in the diagnosis and management of these complications must be present and aware of the problem.

4. These people must be onsite (or immediately available) as long as procedures are being performed and recovering patients are still in the facility.

Inspection of the Products of Conception

At the completion of a first or second trimester evacuation, the physician must be able to assure him- or herself (and the patient) that:

1. The patient is no longer pregnant.

2. No significant fetal or placental tissue has been left in the uterus.

3. There is no continuing pregnancy or ectopic pregnancy present.

These questions are easily and rapidly answerable by the physician (or a designated associate) as soon as the procedure is over and the tissue is examined. It is not safe or prudent to delegate this to a pathologist to be performed one or more days later. The pathologist's assistance is required if there is any question of fetal or placental tissue not being present, if a hydatiform mole or choriocarcinoma is expected, or if suspicion of intra-amniotic infection is being entertained.

The techniques of tissue examination have been outlined in detail by Burnhill et al. (1978), Jerome et al. (1981), Koplik (1980a; 1980b), Munsik (1982), and Lindahl and Ahlgren (1986).

In brief the tissue is:

1. Thoroughly washed in water.

2. Laid out in a dish (preferably transparent with a light source beneath).

3. Reviewed for placenta or fetus using magnification if needed.

If a fetus beyond 10 weeks age is recognized, the fragments should be reassembled to see if the fetus is essentially complete.

A helpful hint is the use of plain white vinegar to make it easier to recognize the placenta in very early gestations. The vinegar washes off the remaining blood and bleaches the villi white. A few minutes devoted to this task will prevent a great many unnecessary repeat procedures for incomplete abortion, hemorrhage, infection, missed ectopic pregnancy, and continuing pregnancy.

Triage of Suspected High-Risk Patients

Not infrequently the clinician may finish a procedure, examine the tissue, or be called to look at the patient in the recovery room and experience a vague (or precise) sense of everything not being all right. Some of these suspicions are triggered by:

1. Heavy bleeding at the onset of dilation or during the procedure.

2. Loss of firmness or tone, enlarging of the cavity, or failure to elicit a "scrape" sound with a sharp curette at the end of the procedure.

3. Prolonged or abnormal pain during the procedure.

4. Scant tissue obtained and inability to delineate placental tissue.

5. Transient or minor changes in the patient's general condition as outlined in the previous section on Patient Monitoring.

When these suspicions are recognized:

1. The patient's chart should be specially marked or logged.

2. Appropriate additional diagnositc or therapeutic measures should be undertaken, such as:

   a. Quantitative hCG.

a. Quantitative HCG.

b. Ultrasound or other radiologic examination.

c. Repeat examination, preferably by a second clinician.

d. Immediate hematocrit, blood for type/Rh, cross matching blood.

e. Initiation of intravenous line.

f. Frequent monitoring of vital signs.

g. Timely transfer to the hospital.

3. Informing the patient (and any accompanying persons) of the nature of the problem or possible problem and of the measures needed to be taken, the reasons for taking them, and the attendant risks.

4. If the problem does not require immediate hospitalization, the facility needs to be assured that the patient's name, address, and telephone number are correct. Additional (confidential) contact information should be sought and follow-up phone calls and facility appointment times made (and recorded).

The person(s) on emergency call should have the appropriate identifying information and suspected problem listed on their on-call log for ease of and rapid identification should a suspected condition (i.e., ectopic pregnancy) move to an emergency situation.

SUMMARY

The broad general principles for preparing for complications of pregnancy termination are outlined.

· Effective risk management requires anticipatory actions to be taken.

· Protocols should be prepared and rehearsed for potential medical, surgical, psychological, and facility problems.

· Equipment should be stocked in an immediately available and clearly identified location.

· Personnel should be acquainted with, trained for, and periodically drilled or rehearsed in the steps to be taken should a problem arise.

REFERENCES

Burnhill, M. S. Physician's Manual, 3rd ed., p. 1. Preterm Institute, Newton, Massachusetts, 1975.

Burnhill, M. S. Reducing the morbidity of vacuum aspiration abortion. International Journal of Gynaecology and Obstetrics 16:204, 1978a.

Burnhill, M. S. Vaginal second trimester abortion. In J. J. Sciarra, G. I. Zatuchni, J. J. Speidel, eds., Risks, Benefits, and Controversies in Fertility Control, p. 331. Harper and Row, Hagerstown, Maryland, 1978b.

Burnhill, M. S. Reducing complications of first-trimester abortion. Contemporary Obstetrics and Gynecology 13:146, 1979a.

Burnhill, M. S. Reducing the morbidity of vacuum aspiration abortion. In G. I. Zatuchni, J. J. Sciarra, J. J. Speidel, eds., Pregnancy Termination, p. 136. Harper and Row, Hagerstown, Maryland, 1979b.

Burnhill, M. S. Risk management in pregnancy termination. In J. J. LaFerla, ed., Clinics in Obstetrics and Gynaecology, p. 145. W. B. Saunders Company, Philadelphia, 1986.

Burnhill, M. S., Armstead, J. S., Kessel, E., et al. Computer-assisted evaluation of demographic trends and morbidity date in first trimester vacuum aspiration. Advances in Planned Parenthood 12(4):212, 1978.

Burnhill, M. S., Danon, M. Dilapan use after 12 weeks of pregnancy. Paper presented at a meeting of the National Abortion Federation, Boston, 1985.

Burnhill, M. S., Edelman, D. A., Armstead, J. S. The relationship between gestational age and the weight of the products of conception. Advances in Planned Parenthood 13(364):9, 1978.

Burnhill, M. S., Robinson, J. C. Dilapan: An improved hydrophilic dilator. Paper presented at a meeting of the National Abortion Federation/Planned Parenthood of America Federation, Atlanta, 1984.

Cates, W., Grimes, D. A. Morbidity and mortality of abortion in the United States. In J. Hodgson, ed., Abortion and Sterilization, Medical and Social Aspects. Academic Press, London, 1981a.

Cates, W., Grimes, D. A. Deaths from second trimester abortion by dilatation and evacuation: Causes, prevention, facilities. Obstetrics and Gynecology 58:401, 1981b.

Darney, P. Abortion: Minimizing risks and complications. Paper presented at the Western Regional Medical Conference, Planned Parenthood Federation of America, San Diego, California, April 12, 1984.

Grimes, D., Cates, W. Complications from legally induced abortion: A review. Obstetrical and Gynecological Survey 34:177, 1979.

Grimes, D., Schulz, K. F., Cates, W. J. Prevention of uterine perforation during curettage abortion. JAMA 251:2108, 1984.

Hern, W. M. Abortion Practice. J. B. Lippincott, Philadelphia, 1981.

Hodgson, J., ed. Abortion and Sterilization: Medical and Social Aspects. Academic Press, London, 1981.

Jerome, M., Armstead, J., Burnhill, M. S., Feller, L. L. Early recognition of ectopic pregnancy at a free-standing abortion clinic. Advances in Planned Parenthood 15(4):144, 1981.

Koplik, L. H. Examination of Tissue. Paper presented at Risk Management Seminar on First Trimester Abortion, Planned Parenthood Federation of America, Session III, Los Angeles, California, February 10, 1980a.

Koplik, L. H. Incomplete and failed abortions, ectopic pregnancies. Paper presented at Risk Management Seminar on First Trimester Abortion, Planned Parenthood Federation of America, Session VII, Los Angeles, California, February 10, 1980b.

LaFerla, J. J., ed. Clinics in Obstetrics and Gynaecology 13(1). W. B. Saunders Company, Philadelphia, 1986.

Lindahl, B., Ahlgren, M. Identification of chorion villi in abortion specimens. Obstetrics and Gynecology 67(1):79, 1986.

McIntosh, K. Quality Assurance Program--A Manual. Planned Parenthood Federation of America, New York, 1984.

Munsick, R. A. Clinical test for placenta in 300 consecutive menstrual aspirations. Obstetrics and Gynecology 60(6):738, 1982.

Oliva, G. Quality Assurance in an abortion program. Paper presented at Risk Management Quality Assurance Seminar, Planned Parenthood Federation of America, Los Angeles, California, December 1, 1980.

Peterson, H. B., Grimes, D. A., Cates, W., et al. Comparative risk of death from induced abortion at 12 weeks gestation performed with local versus general anesthesia. American Journal of Obstetrics and Gynecology 19:155, 1981.

Schulz, K. F., Grimes, D. A., Cates, W. Measures to prevent cervical injury during suction curettage abortion. Lancet i:1182, 1983.

Soderstrom, R. M., Burnhill, M. S., Green, P. M. Complications and risk management in reproductive health. Paper presented at the Annual Meeting of the Association of Planned Parenthood Professionals, Los Angeles, California, November 1, 1984.

Stubblefield, P. Current technology for abortion. Current Problems in Obstetrics and Gynecology 11(4):33, 1979.

Zatuchni, G. I., Sciarra, J. J., Speidel, J. J., eds. Pregnancy Termination, Procedures, Safety, and New Developments. Harper and Row, Hagerstown, Maryland, 1979.

PROBLEM OF SEPTIC ABORTION IN BANGLADESH AND

THE NEED FOR MENSTRUAL REGULATION

Syeda Firoza Begum

M.B.B.S., F.R.C.O.G.
Professor and Head
Department of Obstetrics and Gynecology
Dhaka Medical College & Hospital

President
Bangladesh Association for the Prevention
    of Septic Abortion (BAPSA)
Dhaka, Bangladesh

Khalid Jalil

M.B.B.S., Assistant Registrar
Dhaka Medical College & Hospital
Dhaka, Bangladesh

INTRODUCTION

The legal provision governing the practice of induced abortion in Bangladesh is very restricted; termination of pregnancy is not allowed except to save the life of the mother (Bhiwandiwala, 1982). The revolutionary changes towards liberalization of laws allowing performance of abortion in many countries of the world during the decades of the 1960s and 1970s have not yet influenced the legal structure of Bangladesh (Lee, 1973). Abortions are known to be performed in many countries despite the existing legal status, liberal or restricted. As estimated in 1980, about 30 to 55 million abortions were performed annually throughout the world, of which about half were illegal (Liskin, 1980). Until recently there was very little knowledge about the rate and pattern of induced abortion in Bangladesh and its health implications. Generally, the practice of induced abortion was believed to be very infrequent and socially condemned. There was also some social stigma attached to the procedure, because the need for pregnancy termination was mostly perceived, in a cultural sense, as a clandestine solution to out-of-wedlock pregnancies.

HOSPITAL ADMISSION FOR ABORTION

In the mid 1970s, it was acknowledged for the first time that a large proportion of hospital admissions in the obstetric units of the large hospitals were for management of complication of abortion, a large portion illegally induced. This awareness led to a number of hospital abortion studies during 1977 to 1979. Results of such studies in three hospitals showed that reportedly 17.8 percent of the patients admitted for abortion complication were induced before admission

(Table 1) (Jabeen, 1980). The proportion of induced abortion was highest in the Dhaka Medical Hospital (24.5 percent). Circumstantial evidence drawn from the study, however, led to a suspicion that an unknown, but perhaps substantial, proportion of reportedly spontaneous abortion cases were also, in fact, induced. They were reported as spontaneous because of the illegal status of induced abortion. The same study also revealed the commonly used methods of inducing abortion (Table 2). Introduction of solid objects in the cervical canal was found to be the most frequently used method (42.2 percent), followed by use of oral abortifacients (35.1 percent). Interestingly, the method of abortion induction varied between hospitals. For example, use of solid objects was 32.3 percent in the Dhaka Medical College Hospital, 96.4 percent in Sir Salimullah Medical College Hospital and 61.7 percent in Chittagong Medical College Hospital. These variations are partially explained by the fact that each of these hospitals serve different groups of the population which vary in their socio-cultural patterns. For example, the Dhaka Medical Hospital serves more urban middle-class people, the Salimullah Hospital serves more slum and semi-rural people, and the Chittagong Hospital serves a combination of rural and some urban commercial people.

Another report based on an analysis of data from Dhaka Medical College Hospital alone (Table 3) showed that, of the total 491 women admitted for complication of induced abortion, 49 percent were induced by a non-medical person,

Table 1: Percentage Distribution of Abortion Admissions by Type of Abortion and Hospital

Abortion Type	DMCH (N = 1022)	SSMCH (N = 998)	Ctg. MCH (N = 605)	Total (N = 3625)
Induced outside	24.5	5.7	15.7	17.8
Spontaneous	75.4	94.3	84.3	82.1
Induced in hospital	0.1	0.0	0.0	0.1

Notes: DMCH = Dhaka Medical College Hospital; SSMCH = Sir Salimullah Medical College Hospital; Ctg. MCH = Chittagong Medical College Hospital.
Source: Jabeen, 1980.

Table 2: Distribution of Induced Abortion Cases by Method of Initiation of Abortion

Method of Initiation	DMCH (N = 492)	SSMCH (N = 56)	Ctg. MCH (N = 94)	Total (N = 642)
Chemical Installation	6.1	0.0	2.1	5.0
Solid objects	32.3	96.4	61.7	42.2
Oral abortifacients	41.7	3.6	19.2	35.1
Dilatation	7.9	0.0	3.2	6.5
Other	12.0	0.0	13.8	11.2

Source: Adapted from Jabeen, 1980.

Table 3: Distribution of Hospital Abortions
in DMCH by Type of Practitioner

Type of Practitioner	Percentage
Nonmedical	49
Paramedical	28
Physician	14
Self	8
Other	1
Total	100

Source: Khan et al., 1984.

28 percent by paramedial personnel like a nurse, midwife, or family welfare visitors, 14 percent by a physician, and 8 percent were self-induced (Khan, 1984).

COMPLICATION

Of the reported 491 women admitted to the DMCH for induced abortion, about half (49.7 percent) had at least some complication (Table 4). About a quarter (24.5 percent) had sepsis along with other complications like uterine perforation, cervical laceration, or excessive bleeding, and 14.6 percent had sepsis alone. About 11 percent had excessive bleeding without any sepsis. Thirty-eight women (9.7 percent) died and 11 required total hysterectomy. The women who died were younger in age, less educated, had fewer live births and were more likely to come from a slum dwelling background. Nearly all the women who died (94.7 percent) had the procedure initiated by a non-medical person.

DRAIN ON HOSPITAL RESOURCE

The study under discussion also showed that a substantial amount of hospital resources were consumed for management of induced abortion cases (Table 5). On average, the women needed to stay in the hospital for six days. Those induced by chemical instillation and insertion of solid objects required a longer hospital stay (11.3 and 9.1 days respectively). About a third of the cases required transfusion; again, those induced by chemical instillation and insertion of solid objects required transfusions more frequently (81.1 percent and 52.5 percent, respectively). About 37 percent required therapeutic antibiotics. Although difficult to quantify in monetary terms, it is quite obvious that hospital admissions for illegally induced abortion cases cause a considerable amount of wastage of our hospital resources.

NATIONAL ESTIMATE OF ABORTION MORTALITY

A survey of pregnancy related deaths in Bangladesh in 1978 identified 1933 pregnancy related deaths including 498 due to abortion. Thus, the consequences of induced abortion accounted for about a quarter (25.8 percent) of all maternal deaths (Rochat, 1981). Extrapolating the proportion of maternal deaths caused by induced abortion from the prevailing maternal mortality rate drawn from the Matlab experience, it was estimated that about 7,800 women in Bangladesh died of induced abortion complication in 1978 (Measham, 1981). This survey has documented, at least in part, the magnitude of the overall health problems caused by the practice of illegally induced abortion in the country. Prior to the survey, there was practically no evidence beyond some conjectural assumptions of the rate of induced abortion and its mortality risk.

Table 4: Distribution of Induced Abortion Cases
in DMCH by Types of Complications

Complication		Percentage
No complication		50.3
Complications		49.7
sepsis and other	24.5	
sepsis only	14.6	
other	10.6	
Total		100.0
Total number		491

Source: Khan et al., 1984.

Table 5: Distribution of Complications (excluding sepsis) and Hospital
Resources Used, by Method of Induction of Abortion (%)

Complications and Hospital Resources	Total	Method of Abortion				
		Chemical Instilla- tion	Insertion of Solid Objects	Dilation and/or Evacuation	Oral Aborti- facients	Menstrual Regula- tion
Complications						
None	64.8	31.6	38.7	60.5	86.8	91.5
Uterine perforation	8.4	5.3	22.7	2.6	0.0	0.0
Cervical laceration	2.6	1.6	6.7	0.0	0.5	0.0
Excess blood loss	23.6	60.5	30.1	36.8	12.7	8.5
Other	0.6	0.0	1.8	0.0	0.0	0.0
Total	100.0	100.0	100.0	100.0	100.0	100.0
No. of women	491	38	163	38	204	47
Hospital Resource						
Mean hospitali- zation time (days)	6.0	11.3	9.1	4.5	3.7	2.4
% receiving transfusions	33.5	81.1	52.5	34.2	16.2	4.3
% receiving therapeutic antibiotics	36.9	91.9	78.5	26.3	3.9	0.0

Source: Khan et al., 1984.

A more recent survey conducted in two Upazilas of Bangladesh in 1982-83, found an induced abortion ratio of 44.2 per 1000 live births and a death-to-case rate of 2.4 percent of induced abortion (Table 6) (Khan, 1985). Applying these rates to the total population of Bangladesh estimated at 94.7 million in 1983, the estimated number of induced abortion performed in Bangladesh during that time period would have been 163,244. There were reasons to suggest that the induced abortion ratio in the survey was subject to underreporting, which would also render the number of induced abortions an underestimate. Presuming that the estimated induced abortion deaths of 7,800 in 1978 also occurred in 1983, an alternative estimate of the number of induced abortions in the country would be 325,000 which can be derived by applying the induced abortion mortality risk of 2.4 percent to the estimated total of induced abortion deaths of 7,800 in 1978.

The evidence suggests that the practice of induced abortion along with the resultant mortality risk gives rise to a magnitude of health problems.

ROLE OF MENSTRUAL REGULATION

Use of menstrual regulation (MR) can play an important role in the improvement of maternal health by substituting MR for the practice of induced abortion performed under unsanitary and clandestine conditions. MR was introduced in Bangladesh in several clinical settings and on a more organized scale in the Mohammadpur Model Clinic in 1974. Since its introduction, MR has been steadily gaining popularity. There are indications that the provision of MR services has given the concerned clinics the credibility by which the clinics were able to develop a sustained high level of overall contraceptive acceptance.

The effect of MR services is already reflected in the fact that after introduction of MR services in the neighborhood, abortion-related hospital admissions in the large hospitals have shown signs of decline. Table 7 shows the number of induced abortion admissions in DMCH for different years (Dhaka Medical College, 1984), indicating a downward trend of all abortion admissions from 19.6 percent during 1977-1978, 16.3 percent in 1979-1980, to 10.6 percent each in 1981-1982 and 1983-1984.

Table 6: Number and Rate of Maternal Deaths, Induced Abortion and Septic and Induced Abortion Death Rate, September 1982 to August 1983

Event	Number	Ratio per 1,000 Live Births	Percent of All Maternal Deaths	Death-to-Case Rate As % of All Induced Abortions
Live births	9,317	--	--	--
Induced abortion	412	44.2		
Maternal death	58	6.2		
Septic abortion death	12	1.3	20.7	
Induced abortion deaths	10	1.1	17.2	2.4

Source: Khan, et al., 1985.

Table 7: Number and Percentage of Admission in DMCH for Management of
Spontaneous and Induced Abortion Complications, 1975–1984

Year	Spontaneous Abortion		Induced Abortion		Total	
	No.	%	No.	%	No.	%
1975–76	2,050	84.7	370	15.3	2,420	100.0
1977–78	2,052	80.4	500	19.6	2,552	100.0
1979–80	2,146	83.7	418	16.3	2,564	100.0
1981–82	2,360	89.4	279	10.6	2,639	100.0
1983–84	2,537	89.4	302	10.6	2,839	100.0

ROLE OF MR IN THE FAMILY PLANNING PROGRAM IN BANGLADESH

Although the existing legal provision prohibits termination of pregnancy except in cases required to save the life of the mother, liberal legal interpretation of MR has allowed inclusion of MR in the family planning program and provision of MR services in the government operated clinics (Ali, 1978). The Institute of Law and International Affairs has concluded that ". . . the post-conceptive method of 'menstrual regulation' as a means of birth control does not come under section 312 of the Penal Code. Under statutory schemes, pregnancy is an essential element of the crime of abortion, but the use of menstrual regulation makes it virtually impossible for the prosecutor to meet the required proof, . . . MR is now recognized as an interim method of establishing non-pregnancy for the woman who is at risk of being pregnant. Whether or not she is, in fact, pregnant is no longer an issue" (Ali, 1978).

This scope has been appropriately exploited by the official family planning program to introduce MR throughout the country. For that purpose, large numbers of paramedics and physicians have been trained in the MR procedure, and MR equipment has been supplied to the clinics. By February, 1985, a total of 2238 physicians and 2247 paramedics were trained.

Presently, MR services are available in most family planning clinics under the government program. Table 8 presents the number of yearly MR procedures performed in the country since mid-1970, showing a sharp increase in the late 1970s and early 1980s. The number of MRs performed as presented in Table 8 is perhaps underreported. Private clinics and even government doctors and paramedics performing an MR on a private basis usually do not report such cases.

Government policy is to strengthen MR services through further expansion and improvement in quality. This policy is, however, most seriously jeopardized by restricted funding policies of the donors, particularly USAID and other multinational agencies and intermediary organizations dependent on United States support. This funding restriction precludes provision of MR services in all clinics relying on financial support of such donors.

SUMMARY

The existing penal code in Bangladesh does not permit termination of pregnancy except when necessary to save the life of the mother. Until recently, the practice of induced abortion was believed to be very infrequent and also associated with some degree of social stigma. But there were many admissions in the obstetric units of the hospitals for management of complicated and septic abortions. As a result, a sizeable fraction of the hospital beds of the obstetric units in most large

Table 8: Yearly Performance of MR Procedures
in Bangladesh since 1975

Year	Number of MRs Performed	Index of Increase (1975-1976 = 100
1975-76	4,408	100
1976-77	6,687	151
1977-78	6,135	139
1978-79	4,412	100
1979-80	10,479	238
1980-81	28,041	636
1981-82	42,427	963
1982-83	58,579	1,329
1983-84	56,728	1,280
July 1984 to February 1985	43,870	

Source: MIS Reports, Ministry of Health.

hospitals used to be occupied by women suffering from complications of illegal abortion. It has also been shown that hospital admissions for management of abortion-related complications cause a considerable drain on the hospital resources in terms of medicines, facilities, manpower, and transfusion.

A survey of pregnancy-related deaths in 1978 estimated that 7,800 women died of complications of induced abortion, which accounted for about a quarter of all maternal deaths. A more recent study of maternal mortality in a rural area found an abortion ratio of 44.2 induced abortions per 1,000 live births and a death-to-case rate of 2.4 percent. By applying this finding to the whole country, it was estimated that every year there are at least 163,244 induced abortion cases performed in the country. Applying the induced abortion mortality risk of 2.4 percent to the estimate of 7,800 induced abortion deaths, it can alternately be estimated that about 325,000 induced abortions are performed annually.

This evidence suggests that menstrual regulation (MR) can play a very important role in improving maternal health by substituting for the otherwise unsanitary, clandestine procedure of induced abortion. MR was first introduced in Bangladesh in the early 1970s by the Mohammadpur Model Clinic and a few NGOs. Since its introduction, MR has shown signs of increasing popularity. Family planning clinics providing MR services have developed better credibility, leading to greater acceptance of all family planning methods, whereas clinics without any MR services show poorer performance. The number of admissions resulting from abortion complications declined in both Dhaka Medical College Hospital and Chittagong Medical College Hospital as MR services became available in those areas.

Although the existing penal code prohibits termination of pregnancy except to save the life of the mother, legal interpretation allows menstrual regulation. This scope has been conveniently utilized by gradual introduction of MR, mainly through training of female paramedics and the establishment of services in the clinics.

Presently, MR services are widely available in most family planning clinics. Government efforts to further expand MR facilities are, however, seriously jeopardized by restrictive funding policies of donors, particularly USAID.

REFERENCES

Ali, M. S., Zahir, M., Hassan, K. M. Report on legal aspects of population planning in Bangladesh, The Bangladesh Institute of Law and International Affairs, Dhaka, 1978.

Bhiwandiwala, P. P., Cook, R. J., Dickens, B. M., Polls, M. Menstrual therapies in commonwealth Asian law. International Journal of Gynaecology and Obstetrics 20:273, 1982.

Hospital Records, Obstetrics Department, Dhaka Medical College Hospital. 1975—1984.

Jabeen, S., Nazmul, S., Ahmed, G. A study of the abortion related admission in three hospitals in Bangladesh, BFRP Contributors Conference, Dhaka. 1980.

Khan, A. R., Begum, S. F., Covington, D. L., et al. Risks and costs of illegally induced abortion in Bangladesh, Journal of Bio-social Science 16:89, 1984.

Khan, A. R., Rochat, A. W., Jahan, F. A., et al. Practice of induced abortion in a rural area of Bangladesh, Studies in Family Planning 17:95, 1986.

Lee, L. T. Five largest countries allow legal abortion on broad grounds. Population Report Series F, No. I, Washington, D.C., 1973.

Liskin, L. S. Complications of abortion in developing countries, Population Report Series F, No. 7, Johns Hopkins University, Baltimore, Maryland, 1980.

Measham, A. R., Obaidullah, M., Rosenberg, M. J. Complications from induced abortion in Bangladesh related to types of practitioner and methods, and impact on morbidity. Lancet, January 1981.

Rochat, R. W., Jabeen, S., Rosenberg, M. J., et al. Maternal and abortion related deaths in Bangladesh, 1978-1979. International Journal of Gynaecology and Obstetrics 19:155, 1981.

MENSTRUAL REGULATION SERVICE DELIVERY

Sandra Mostafa Kabir

Executive Director
Bangladesh Women's Health Coalition
Dhaka, Bangladesh

BACKGROUND

The Bangladesh Women's Health Coalition (BWHC) was founded when the Concerned Women for Family Planning's Menstrual Regulation (MR) Unit closed down due to USAID funding restrictions. A dearth of quality women's reproductive health care facilities and practical training opportunities for paramedics were also very pertinent in the decision to set up the Coalition. This organization, an affiliate of the International Women's Health Coalition, consisted of only a tiny office at its inception in April 1980. Now BWHC has a central office, six family planning/Maternal & Child Health clinics, and an income-generating sewing center; provides legal lectures and legal aid to its staff and other women; performs the functions of an employment exchange for women seeking jobs mainly with nongovernmental organizations in the health and family planning sector; and undertakes training of government paramedics called Family Welfare Visitors and staff from various family planning and health agencies. BWHC also has a research and evaluation unit which undertakes baseline surveys, comparison studies, studies on different methods of family planning, and monitoring of clinic performance.

LOCALE AND SERVICES

Our clinics are each unique in their locale. The first clinic established is situated in the old section of Dhaka, the capital of Bangladesh. Another is in the biggest inland port and industrial area; the third is on the outskirts of a district town; a more recently opened clinic is at the small county level which is both rural and industrial; and the newest facility is situated in the deep village where there is no running water, electricity, or gas and which is reached journeying by jeep, country boat, or cycle rickshaw. Services at the clinics are provided mainly by women paramedics with the backup support of part-time doctors and consist of the following:

- Contraceptive counseling
- Menstrual regulation (uterine aspiration)
- Insertion of Copper T IUDs
- Injectable contraceptives (both Depo-provera and Noresthisterate)
- Supply of pills, condoms, and foam
- Referral to governmental or nongovernmental organization clinics for sterilization services

- Basic health care for women and children which includes pre- and postnatal care, diagnosis and treatment of primary illnesses (upper respiratory tract infections, worms, diarrhea, dysentery, scabies, etc.)
- Immunizations for DPT, DT, TT, BCG, measles, and polio
- Referral to government hospitals for treatment of the more complicated diseases
- Group talks or lectures for women on health and family planning related subjects, such as breast-feeding, nutrition, weaning, etc.
- Pathological tests for Hb, albumen, and sugar

CLIENTELE

Because of the different locales of the clinics, the clients are also varied. In the city or town areas the women are predominantly middle class with approximately seven to eight years of schooling. In the rural areas the clients are very poor and invariably illiterate. City women come primarily for family planning services, whereas those in the village areas come initially for the treatment of their children and later for family planning. A comparison of MR client characteristics for the Coalition Clinic, Mirpur, and the Mohammadpur Fertility Services and Training Center (Chowdhury, 1984; Akhter, 1983) shows that most MR clients are between the ages of 25 and 29 years, have received from one to ten years of schooling, and are mainly housewives.

STAFFING

The staffing pattern at each of the BWHC clinics varies somewhat. All clinics have administrators who are responsible for finance, accounts, personnel, and day-to-day operations of each facility. At four of the clinics the administrator is also responsible for counseling both new and old or continuing family planning clients. This step was taken since the government did not approve this category of staff at three of the clinics and at the fourth we have tried to cut back on expenses by amalgamating the position of administrator and counselor. Every clinic has one or two paramedics who are called Family Welfare Visitors. The paramedics graduate after taking an eighteen-month course at the Family Welfare Visitors Training Institutes after completing at least ten years of schooling. The paramedics are assisted by one or two nurses aides who take blood pressure and perform immunizations and basic pathological tests. The part-time doctors are responsible for Maternal and Child Health Care. They diagnose and prescribe medications for clients coming for basic health care and handle the difficult or complicated family planning cases. In addition to this staff, each clinic has two women attendants to keep the premises clean and two guards for security purposes. A major reason why women come to the Coalition clinics is that almost all the staff are women. Socially, this is easily accepted by the predominantly conservative Muslim population. Also, the female staff is generally more caring and understanding of the clients' problems, whether these problems be related to their personal lives, health, or family planning. Two of the clinics have a separate position of counselor whose sole duty is to provide advice, information, and guidance to the family planning clientele. I would like to mention that counseling is a very important aspect of the clinics and much emphasis is put on quality, caring counseling. The six clinics of the BWHC receive backup support from the central office which arranges for their finances, equipment and supplies, staff training, monitoring and evaluation, and regular supervisory visits.

COUNSELING

A major emphasis of the Coalition is the provision of high standard, individualized, and confidential counseling for each family planning client visiting the clinics. This service is provided not only to women but to attending husbands as well.

From the Coalition's experience over the past five years it is apparent that counseling is an all-important part of providing quality family planning services to both women and men. At the Mirpur Clinic, which began service delivery in October 1983, family planning clients received very little counseling because paramedics were too busy providing service delivery and filling out forms. This situation was changed when the clinic administrator was trained in counseling and began providing this service to all family planning clients visiting the clinic. Table 1 shows the percentage increase in adoption of a family planning method after MR at the clinic before and after the administrator was trained in counseling techniques.

Counseling also increased the number of women coming back to the clinic for follow-up services from 11 percent to 37 percent. All the counselors are trained at the Dhaka Clinic, which is the oldest facility and where the administrator-/counselor is experienced, mature and well-suited for the job. Trainees are given booklets to read on family planning methods, counseling and related subjects. They also go through a series of lectures and question-and-answer sessions with the medical staff and observe the training counselor for the first few days. Then the trainee counselors participate in the counseling sessions with the clients and when ready actually undertake counseling under the supervision of the trainer. They either return to the Dhaka Clinic after three or four months or the trainer visits the counselors at the individual clinics for performance review. An important aspect of the BWHC training program is in-service and on-the-job training, which is a regular and continuous process for all staff.

QUALITY SERVICE

The high-quality of services provided by the Coalition Clinics is well known in Bangladesh. This is made possible through training of all staff when they initially join and through continuing in-service courses. Periodic visits by management of the central office for supervision and discussion of problems is another vital aspect of maintaining high quality service. The medical director during her monthly visits to each clinic talks to the staff about any difficulties they may have faced and discusses complications. She makes sure that the medical staff undertakes procedures correctly and arranges for their training when necessary. Orientation at other government or nongovernment clinics are also arranged for our staff so that they can learn new techniques and methods and compare working standards. The paramedics who provide most of the family planning services are not only efficient in their work, but also caring in their attitude towards clients. They can relate very easily with women coming to the clinic and create a wonderful rapport with them. As mentioned earlier, counseling is another important and intrinsic part of quality service. Each and every family planning

Table 1: Percent of Women Accepting Various Contraceptive Methods before (10/83–3/84) and after (12/84–2/85) Introduction of Counseling, Coalition Clinic, Mirpur, Bangladesh

Method Accepted	Before	After
None	34.7%	4.3%
IUD	45.7%	70.7%
Oral Pill	16.3	18.7
Condom	0.6	--
Injectable	2.7	--
Total	100.0%	100.0%

client, whether it is her first or repeat visit, is counseled carefully and all her questions are answered. The clinics offer waiting rooms where the clients have an opportunity to talk with each other and areas where they can talk privately with their husbands or with clinic staff. For example, an MR or IUD client is counseled and then taken to the examination room, where she is helped up onto the examination table. During the procedure, which is typically performed by a paramedic, another member of staff talks to the client to relax and reassure her. After the procedure she is given a private place to lie down and is offered a cup of tea. The caring attitude and attention given to each client in addition to the maintenance of high medical standards are the most important aspects of quality service. Again and again we find that women come to the clinics after hearing about this specialized service from satisfied clients. This is indeed a tribute to the Coalition's activities.

Yet another attribute of the high quality of service at the BWHC clinics is the referral system we have established with the government and nongovernment hospitals and clinics. A client referred from our clinic is given preferential treatment and has better chances of receiving proper attention at these hospitals and clinics than if she went on her own. In addition, whenever possible, community support is developed. The Coalition's village-level clinic was provided accommodation by the chairman of the county level health complex. This was an incentive to clients to utilize this clinic early and in large numbers.

All the clinics have a uniform pattern of record-keeping. Client flow is determined by each clinic, keeping the convenience of the clients and expediency of operation in mind. Monthly, quarterly, and annual reports on clients, services, and accounts are submitted to the central office to be passed on to the funding agencies. Implementation of staff rules and regulations assures the smooth administration of the central office and each individual clinic. The central office maintains total support to the clinics so that their staff can provide services to the clients, unencumbered by concerns for funds, supplies and other items. Staff morale is kept high through regular visits by central office management to the clinics, staff participation in various seminars and workshops, both in-service training and training at other institutions, regular management workshops, distribution of a trimonthly newsletter on overall Coalition activities, and annual get-togethers for clinic staff and visitors.

The Bangladesh Women's Health Coalition's strong emphasis on quality care results in many benefits:

a) Contraceptive acceptance and use is higher at the Coalition Clinics in comparison to similar clinics which provide both family planning and maternal and child health services.

b) Our clinics, while providing services at a high quality, are also cost effective; on average, at all six clinics each service costs U.S.$0.82 and each client approximately U.S.$1.06.

c) Since high medical and counseling standards are maintained the clinics serve as training centers for doctors, paramedics, counselors, and other clinical personnel who work with either the government or nongovernment organizations.

d) The clinics serve as an example of quality, cost-effective, and well-managed services in Bangladesh to other organizations and to the government.

SERVICE FEES

At the Dhaka Clinic and Narayanganj Clinic (Narayanganj is an inland port and industrialized area) the Coalition charges for services on a sliding-scale basis ranging from free-of-cost up to maximum charge set for each service. These two clinics earn 50 percent of their monthly operating costs from service fees. Charging for service or registration is a unique aspect of the Coalition clinics and affects the type of client coming to the clinics. Poorer women who hear about charges frequently do not even come to the clinic to enquire if free services would be provided. They go to government or other nongovernment organization facilities which in theory are free of cost. The other four Coalition clinics charge only a very nominal registration fee (equivalent to approximately U.S. 3 cents) for each client per visit. Gradually clients are realizing that spending a small amount for quality service is worthwhile and the number of clients is increasing as a result. The average person in Bangladesh is used to a system of free health and family planning services by both the government and nongovernment organizations. When the Coalition clinics first opened there was considerable resentment that even nominal fees were charged, and occasionally accusations were made that staff was pocketing the money. Charging for service depends on educating the population that Bangladesh cannot depend forever on foreign assistance, that every citizen should contribute whatever he or she can towards the cost of services, and that quality services are worth paying for. Except for private practitioners, with which the Coalition has to compete, all other facilities provide free services (although at lower standards). Those clients who come to our clinics and who have sufficient funds often make generous donations in appreciation of our services.

FIELD PROGRAM

One of the weaknesses of our program has been the lack of an organized field program. The Coalition has had to depend on the government and other voluntary organizations to refer clients to the clinics. In addition, follow-up has not been as thorough as it could have been since we have no field workers to visit the homes of the clients who have not come back for a checkup. Outreach workers could find out why women have been unable to come back for a checkup, and actually bring the clients along to the clinic. In the city areas this absence of outreach does not affect the program as much as it does in the rural areas. As of September 1, 1985, funding for outreach programs has been arranged and after sufficient training field workers will be going into the surrounding areas of the clinics to motivate clients and to encourage proper follow-up.

GOVERNMENT SUPPORT AND COOPERATION

The Government of Bangladesh must accord approval for all projects, including those of the BWHC. It provides all contraceptives used in the clinics and a small quantity of medicines for maternal and child health activities. The Coalition also receives free supplies of vaccines and equipment from the Expanded Program for Immunization, which is a government program. Regular monthly and annual performance reports are sent by BWHC to the government at both local and national levels. Cooperation with other nongovernmental voluntary organizations is varied. For example, we provide family planning services and immunizations to a women's sewing center at Dhaka and some nongovernmental organizations bring or refer clients to our clinics. Our influence over referral is limited since most family planning programs receive funds from U.S. government sources and cannot be involved in abortion or related activities. The Coalition is a member of the Voluntary Health Services Society through which coordination and cooperation is extended in seminars, workshops, and training related to both health and family planning.

SUMMARY

The Bangladesh Women's Health Coalition is an organization run by women for women. Its philosophy is to provide high-quality family planning and basic health care services to women and children by a highly trained, motivated, and committed staff. We envision that similar services can and will be started in Bangladesh and other developing countries using the Coalition as an example and impetus.

REFERENCES

Akhter, H. H. Menstrual regulation versus contraception in Bangladesh: Characteristics of the acceptors, Part 1. Studies in Family Planning 14(12):318, 1983.

Chowdhury, G. A. A Study on Sociodemographic Characteristics of 300 MR Clients in Mirpur Coalition Clinic, Dhaka, October 1983—March 1984. Lalmatia, Dhaka, October 1984.

THE KARMAN SYRINGE IN FAMILY PRACTICE:

TECHNIQUES, SAFETY, AND USAGE

Kotha Pannikar

Kedah Klinik
Alor Setar, West Malaysia

I am a Family Physician who provides total health care in addition to abortion services, and was introduced to the Karman Syringe by the late Professor I. S. Puvan, a Tietze disciple, in August 1974. These two great physicians had a vision of making termination of pregnancy available to all women who needed it, not just those who could afford it. To this end, the procedure had to be safe, effective, inexpensive, easily available, and acceptable to women of various cultures and socioeconomic groups. Menstrual regulation (MR) in family practice is the appropriate solution. Let us look at the types of Karman syringes available. The first one did not have a pinch valve; the second one had a rubber bung and a valve which works quite well, but when the rubber bung deteriorates and swells when creating the vacuum, it slips off the plunger with a loud noise. Next came the syringe with a nitrile ring which is excellent for use with first trimester procedures. The fourth generation syringe has a double valve and adaptors for larger cannulae which can be used for late first and early second trimester procedures.

Several steps are necessary to make MR a safe and effective procedure within a family practice.

SELECTION OF CLIENT

Anyone with uncontrolled thyrotoxics, cardiac failure, arrhythmias, obvious blood dyscrasias, or similar unstable conditions should be sent to a well-equipped hospital.

HISTORY

This should include (1) age; (2) L.M.P. [Was it normal? (Clients often report falsely low periods or amenorrhea)]; (3) parity (nullips sometimes claim to be parous); (4) past history of post-partum hemorrhage or retained placenta; (5) past contraceptive use, type of method, and problems, if any.

CONTRACEPTIVE MOTIVATION

Studies have shown that women are more likely to accept contraception after an abortion than at other times. MR should be presented only as a back-up for failed contraception. Contraceptive counseling should allay fears and dismiss myths and old wives' tales. Health benefits to mother and child, and the factors that affect the child's mental development need to be stressed. The woman should be helped to develop a sense of self-worth and self-esteem.

EXAMINATION

Part of the general examination are instructions to empty bladder, taking temperature, blood pressure, and a urine sample to detect sugar and albumin. Goals of the gynecological exam with the speculum are to check for cervical infection, erosion, and state of the os (nulliparous or open). During the bimanual exam, the physician checks uterine size, position, anomalies, tenderness, and looks for adnexal pathology.

PREMED (given 1/2 hour before procedure)

Preoperative medications include: (1) Prophylactic Cotrimoxazole (if any serious allergic reaction occurs it will be while the patient is still in the clinic); if GC, chlamydia, or trichomoniasis infections are seen, therapy is started with a loading dose; (2) Valium, 2 mg orally; (3) Avomine, if less than 8 weeks L.M.P.; (4) Stelazine, 2 mg if more than 8 weeks L.M.P.

BASIC REQUIREMENTS

1. A clean room with running water to clean instruments.

2. A light source--anglepoise lamp on a stool.

3. The M.R. kit.

4. The table (it can be inexpensive, made by a local carpenter).

5. The sterile tray containing

   a. Graves self-retaining speculum.
   b. Sponge forceps to clean cervix and sponge after procedure.
   c. Pot with two sterile tampons.
   d. One set each of 4-, 5-, and 6-mm cannulae.
   e. Hegar dilators 4 & 5.
   f.* A 6-mm tip ovum forcep to remove products of conception (POC).
   g. Splinter forceps to remove POC from blocked cannulae.

6.* Emergency tray: 2 sterile plastic syringes, 1 Amp. Syntocinon 5 U./ml., 1 Amp. Adona (Carbozochrome sod. sulfonate), 1 Amp. Solucortef, 1 Amp. Adrenalin 1/1000.

7. One dish to empty POC into.

8. One sterile kidney dish with cooled boiled water to clean syringe.

PREPARATION OF THE WOMAN

1. Empty bladder.

2. Position client on the table in lithotomy position with her feet drawn up to her buttocks.

3. While inserting the speculum and cleaning the cervix, the woman is told that she will feel everything, which will be uncomfortable but not painful; that

when nearly finished, the uterus will contract and she will feel an ache in her lower abdomen; that the procedure will be over in less than 5 minutes. Providing this information helps establish a positive attitude.

PROCEDURE

1. The cervix is cleaned with Hibitane in spirit on the tip of a gauze tampon. (If it is dripped into the vagina it will sting.)

2. The tenaculum is applied horizontally on anterior lip of cervix.

3. The cannula is selected and inserted with the following guidelines in mind: 4 mm for nulliparous or less than 6 weeks L.M.P., 5 mm for 6–8 weeks L.M.P., 6 mm for more than 8 weeks L.M.P.

4. A vacuum is created in the syringe and the cannula attached, the thumb lock is released, followed by aspiration and rotation of the cannula to a full 360 degrees.

5. The syringe is emptied into the dish, then flushed with the cooled boiled water. The vacuum is recreated and the procedure continued until grating is felt through a 360-degree turn.

6. The cannula and tenaculum are removed, the tenaculum site is checked for bleeding, and the cervix is cleaned as before.

7. Products of conception are checked to see if the volume of aspirate matches the dates. (Ectopic pregnancy should be considered if it does not correspond.) POC are floated in water to verify villi present. Any suspicious material is sent for histopathology.

POST MR

Medication

1. Trimethoprin-sulfasoxazole or other appropriate antibiotic if infected.

2. Ergonovine tab x 2 days in case of flabby uterus or fibroids, or if the woman has to travel beyond the local area.

3. Oral contraceptives are given to be started on the third day after the procedure. The purpose is to bring on menstruation in 4 weeks and to control the bleeding that will otherwise occur form the third day onwards.

   Instructions to the patient are to abstain from coitus for 2 weeks and to return to the clinic if she is still bleeding after 5 days; if she experiences any abdominal pain (she may have an ectopic pregnancy or PID); if she has no period at the end of the first cycle of oral contraceptives.

COMPLICATIONS

· Pain, especially in nullips or non-gravid women, is relieved by Ponstan or other mild analgesics

· Vomiting--some women vomit with uterine contraction. They are given special care and support.

· Syncope, especially if the patient has fasted.

- Perforation--in 14,700 we had one anterior perforation that required hospitalization and laparotomy. That was the 1,445th MR procedure done by the same operator.

- Incomplete aspiration because POC in left cornu, tight internal os, done under general anaesthesia.

- Twinning--5 in our series, the last one in a double uterus, 1 in each side.

- Ectopic--we have had 5 so far.

- PID--1 in the series. The woman did not take her prophylactic septrin tab as they looked like panadols and she did not have any pain. (We now use capsules.)

- Bleeding tendencies--if the aspirate does not coagulate in the dry dish, give Adona.

- Sensitivity to Septrin--we had three such cases. One went on to a Stevens-Johnson Syndrome and required prolonged steroid therapy. For the other two solucortef was given.

- Very speedy return to fertility if contraception is not started immediately.

- Amenorrhea--This usually happens in women who were not gravid at MR. If oral contraceptives do not work, I use ethinyl estradiol plus orethindrone serially for one or two cycles. I do not know if true Ascherman's syndrome occurs with MR. I have not had one yet.

COST EFFECTIVENESS

With proper care the cannulae easily last for 50 MRs. Maneuvering around the cervical fibroids damages the cannulae. The rubber bungs last for 100 MRs before they start to pop and the rubber washers of the pinch valve last between 200 and 250 MRs. As for the nitrile rings, it is not known how long they last. One has been used for 7,270 MRs and it is still in good condition. We disagree that the type of lubricant used does not affect the life of the syringe. We use silicone grease on the dry syringe, before it is assembled in the morning and dismantle, wash, dry, and apply a drop of silicone liquid on the bung or nitrile ring in the evening. Between procedures, the syringes and cannulae are rinsed with plain tap water. The cannulae are sterilized in Hibitane in spirit 1:10. We do not use Betadine solution as it discolors the cannulae.

CONCLUSION

In conclusion, we are convinced that the Karman syringe is a very important piece of equipment in primary health care. Other than its use in the treatment of failed contraception, it can also be used:

1. To bring down a lost IUD thread.

2. To do a diagnostic curettage (biopsy).

3. To treat an incomplete abortion.

4. To treat a missed abortion.

5. To treat septic abortion after institution of antibiotic theraphy. It is much safer than using the curette on an inflamed and pregnant (thus very soft) uterus.

6.   To treat molar pregnancies.

7.   To treat dysfunctional uterine bleeding.

The savings to the government health care programs would be monumental if one takes into account the savings in staff time, operating theater time, and hospital bed occupancy. To the patient, as no anaesthetic is given, the anaesthetic risk is obviated. Also, no arrangements need be made to care for the family while the patient is in hospital. An outpatient procedure assures confidentiality as the woman's visit could easily have been for a headache or constipation as for an abortion. If asked to name three health boons to womankind in this century, I would answer: contraception, the Pap smear, and the Karman syringe.

TRAINING IN MENSTRUAL REGULATION:

THE PHILIPPINE EXPERIENCE

Lydia Aznar Alfonso

Chairman, Department of Family Planning
Southwestern University College of Medicine
Cebu City, The Philippines

INTRODUCTION

The Philippines with its 54 million inhabitants, is 80 percent Catholic and 15 percent belong to various sects or denominiations which oppose abortion in any form. Abortion is illegal and the government is straightforward in its policy statement for the Philippine population program: "all acceptable methods of contraception, except abortion, will be provided for acceptors to choose from." Pregnancy termination, even as a back-up method for contraceptive failure, is not acceptable. This policy exists despite our findings in 1980 that contraceptive effectiveness was only around 71 percent, while the contraceptive prevalence rate was estimated at 41 percent.

It is this strong religious influence that has prevented our government from pursuing a more aggressive population program. Our laws are similarly influenced by these religious overtones so that abortion in any form, including menstrual regulation (MR), is a felonious crime looked down on by all sectors of the Philippine society. Also, our culture, deeply rooted in Catholicism, likewise prohibits any discussion about abortion as it carries with it "hiya"--that Filipino trait of shame and guilt.

These religious, legal and cultural barriers have led to increasing problems of unwanted pregnancies, illegal abortions and their morbidity and mortality complications.

In a predominantly Catholic country, the pro-life movement, especially from the religious sectors, exerts pressure on the government and the public to take action against abortion. As a result, those who do provide abortion services always face the threat of harassment, rejection and persecution by the authorities, and society at large. But in spite of the dangers of illicit abortion, the anti-abortion laws, the pro-life movement and cultural considerations, abortion clinics and traditional abortion practitioners who use herbs, abdominal massage or catheters, continue to exist and even prosper in the Philippines.

Statistics from three public hospitals in Metro Manila alone show that about 10−16 percent of the hospital beds in the obstetrics and gynecological wards were occupied by septic cases. The Philippine health statistics in 1979 indicated that around 9 percent of maternal deaths could be attributed to such abortions. However, there is reason to believe that the national health statistics do not reflect the true situation. Since the subject is considered taboo, abortion-related data are not easily accessible.

It was in this kind of environment in early 1980, that a group of concerned women and men decided to organize themselves and respond to the lack of a holistic approach to women's welfare, particularly in addressing the needs of women faced with unwanted and unplanned pregnancies. With help from the Population Crisis Committee and the International Women's Health Coalition, this group of men and women established a non-profit organization.

In the early days trainees were recommended by personal friends of the organizers and consisted of both midwives and medical practitioners. At that time no attempts were made to recruit outside the organizers circle of friends because of the prevailing legal and socio-cultural climate.

The training approach used then was largely tutorial and lasted a month. Trainees observed a number of MR procedures during the first couple of weeks and then performed eight to ten procedures with supervision. The training manual developed by the International Women's Health Coalition was of great use to the trainees. They were given refresher courses on family planning and sexually transmitted diseases and received training in counseling, staff-client relationships, and in community organization techniques. The latter was to enable them to conduct information and education activities in the community where their clinics were located. It was only after gaining some measure of stability in its operations that the organization felt it was ready to expand its services to the provinces.

A consultative workshop with MR service providers was convened to discuss and comment on the proposed MR training curriculum, the distribution system for MR kits and related commodities, and the organizational requirements for setting up an MR community-based service program. The recommendations were used in finalizing the design of the MR/CBS program for the Philippines, which will be implemented in some provinces where the effectiveness and usefulness of the design will be tested.

THE TRAINING PROGRAM

An organization or a coordinating body has to conduct and assess the needs of the country for MR service, review the existing health facilities, personnel and available finances.

The training institution or center should be identified, along with the available trainers and the trainers' qualifications. There should be guidelines for the selection of trainees, course content, certifications after the course and follow-up of trainees.

Ways should be explored in which MR services could be included into the existing health services and family planning clinics, and into the medical or nursing curriculum of an existing medical or nursing school.

The political, legal, religious and cultural constraints in the community should be taken into consideration. Regions of the country where such services will be greatly needed should be identified.

Requirements of a Training Institution

The training center could be located in a university based, hospital based, rural or urban clinic. The following are needed for training:

1. Facilities and equipment--not only for the procedure but also for the treatment of any complications that may arise.

2. Experienced and qualified training staff.

3. Presence of adequate lecture rooms.

4. Facilities for counseling clients and the pre-operative evaluation of clients.

5. Teaching aids such as slides, video films and models.

6. An adequate number of patients to be able to support the training activities of the trainees in the training period.

Trainers' Qualifications

1. Knowledge of different methods of contraception.

2. Experience in surgery and ability to manage complications.

3. Knowledge in analgesia and anesthesia.

4. Knowledge in counseling.

5. Teaching ability including effective communication skills.

6. Knowledge in clinic management.

7. Interest in furthering his or her education and training.

Selection of Trainees Should Include the Following Criteria

1. Willingness to learn and understand.

2. Commitment to the program.

3. Basic knowledge in anatomy, physiology and family planning methods.

4. Sufficient background and ability to do internal examinations. This should be carefully evaluated as accurate assessment of the gestational age appears to be an important factor in reducing risk.

5. Knowledge in national vital statistics and contraceptive prevalence.

The Training Curriculum and Methodology

The objective is to train health professionals to perform safe MR procedures. The training course should include:

1. Orientation on MR and a community-based service program including the concern, goals and objectives of the MR/CBS program as well as the sponsoring organization. The trainees should become familiar with the approaches and strategies employed when introducing MR into their clinics and area of operations. There should be an opportunity to discuss the trainees' and the trainers' expectations from each other.

2. The health and population rationale for the use of MR.

3. Current status of family planning in the country.

4. Reproductive physiology and anatomy.

5. Methods of contraception.

6. Counseling to motivate clients to use more effective contraceptive methods.

7. Preoperative evaluation.

8. Asepsis.

9. Analgesia, anesthesia and resuscitation.

10. Preoperative instructions.

11. MR Technique.

The theoretical portion of MR techniques should be discussed and presented through slides and film presentations. The development and progress of pregnancy may be discussed here. After the theoretical portion, it would be helpful to familiarize the trainees with the MR equipment and give them a feeling for how it works prior to its actual use. The number of procedures to be observed prior to actually preforming a procedure would depend on the trainees' previous medical and family planning experience. The number of procedures required for each trainee greatly depends on the trainees own level of confidence and background.

The practicum portion of MR should be interspersed with discussions of topics also considered important in the implementation of MR/CBS programs. One of these is the legal implication of performing MRs, since abortion is illegal in this country. Trainees should be made aware of the possible risks they may encounter in the course of program implementation and be taught about safeguards and ways of minimizing these risks. The trainees also will be informed about the establishment of a legal fund for MR practitioners. Through this legal fund, MR practitioners will be assured of financial and professional help should they find themselves in a legal bind as long as the organization is assured that policies and minimum requirements for the provision of MR were adhered to.

12. Care and maintenance of MR and related equipment to prolong their use.

13. Complications and their management.

14. Postoperative care. Trainees should understand the importance of reassuring the patient and making her feel at ease and secure. They should also watch for signs and symptoms which would indicate certain complications.

15. Follow-up. The patient is instructed to report to the office after one week or immediately following symptoms of pain and fever and profuse bleeding. The patient must also be given postoperative instructions.

16. Recording and reporting. The importance of maintaining both medical and administrative records should be emphasized.

17. Information and Education. Trainees need to learn how to organize and conduct information and education activities in the community to help the community develop a more responsible attitude toward fertility and sexuality. Information should include women's health, nutrition, sanitation and contraceptive methods to counteract misconceptions and to motivate clients, especially MR clients, to accept more effective methods of contraception.

18. Administration of the clinic. The trainees need to understand the scope of their jobs, their own work load to make services efficient and the duties and responsibilities of each staff in the clinic. A fee structure which will make the service affordable should also be observed. The availability of MR equipment and related commodities should be discussed here.

TEACHING

Teaching aids are needed to reinforce didactic lectures. In addition to lectures, there should be discussions and demonstrations for practical training. The trainees should participate in selecting, counseling, and preparing the patient for MR, the procedure itself and postoperative follow-up. They should be able to assist and perform the procedure under supervision.

The duration of training and number of procedures performed by the trainee depend on the trainee's background. Trainees usually perform 10 procedures or less.

CERTIFICATION

The evaluation and certification of trainees should be based on an evaluation of skills and competency with the procedure itself and such other activities as screening of clients, counseling, analgesia and postoperative care. Trainees could also be evaluated with pre- and post-training testing.

FOLLOW-UP

After 6 months of practice on their own, the performance of the trainees can be evaluated by a team from the head office to determine their level of competence and ability to provide the various services under the MR/CBS program.

REFERRAL SYSTEMS

Establishing a referral network in the areas where MR services are provided is essential. It allows the practitioner in the area to refer difficult cases, promote services in the clinic and to provide support and mutual assistance.

RESEARCH NEED

In order to effectively meet the reproductive health needs of women, much needed areas of research are:

1. Studying the psychological effects of MR on the Filipino woman, finding ways of helping her cope with the negative effects and of motivating her to use more effective contraceptive methods.

2. Studying the extent of the current pregnancy termination situation in the Philippines, including practices, methods used and consequences. Such a study would allow us to develop appropriate approaches in the use of MR as a contraceptive alternative. For example, the study could provide data on the network of untrained abortion practitioners and information on morbidity following illegal abortion.

CONCLUSIONS

It takes time to develop a proper training program which suits the country's needs. We need to constantly revise our assessment and modify our training programs as the situation demands. Success in the implementation of the MR service and training will depend on the political, legal, religious and cultural acceptability of the method, an effective information and education campaign through the radio and other media, the availability and accessability of facilities, and the health personnel's competence in performing the procedure.

Guidelines for training are necessary in order to insure safe and quality services. The MR procedure must be promoted in the Philippines where the services are needed, especially in rural areas where either no contraceptive methods or no effective contraceptives are available.

REFERENCES

Cook, R., Senanayake, P. (eds.). The human problem of abortion. Medical and legal dimensions. IPPF Medical Bulletin, February, p. 12, 1978.

Gallen, M. Abortion Practices in the Philippines: An Exploratory Study Among Clients and Practitioners, Circa 1979. A Research project sponsored by the International Committee on Applied Research in Population (ICARP), May 1980.

Gallen, M. Abortion choices in the Philippines. Journal of Biosocial Science 2(3):281, 1979.

Maranon, A., et al. Compiled Studies on Voluntary Interruption of Pregnancy (VIP) in the Philippines: 1978–1982, (Mimeo), A Joint Research of the Menstrual Regulation and Fertility Center and Southern Mindanao Agricultural Research Center of the University of Southern Mindanao, April 1983.

Valenzuela, A. V. Abortion in Filipino women: Phase I--abortion in a Philippine municipality, Sta. Rosa, Laguna. Journal of the Philippine Medical Association 46:655, 1970.

Valenzuela, A. V., Jara, I. D. Abortion in two Philippine hospitals. Journal of the Philippine Medical Association 54 (11/12):379, Nov.–Dec. 1978.

Valenzuela, et al. Pregnancy Termination Study in Philippine Hospitals in Five Health Regions, Metro Manila: Population Center Foundation, 1982.

DELIVERY OF ABORTION CARE IN THE UNITED STATES

Jacqueline D. Forrest

Director of Research
The Alan Guttmacher Institute
New York, New York, U.S.A.

INTRODUCTION

Shortly after the United States Supreme Court in 1973 legalized abortion nationwide, Christopher Tietze collaborated with The Alan Guttmacher Institute (AGI) in developing and fielding a survey of abortion providers to ascertain the number of abortions and the extent of service accessibility across the country. The AGI Abortion Provider Survey was conducted annually covering the periods 1973–1978 and biannually for years 1979–1982. The 1984–1985 Survey is currently in progress.

The yearly survey data clearly show that since 1973 (see Henshaw, Forrest, Blaine, 1984), abortions have become almost entirely outpatient procedures, most of which occur in freestanding nonhospital clinics. This change occurred for a number of reasons, including reluctance of hospital providers to offer abortion services, improved technology and experience showing nonhospital procedures to be safe, of lower cost and greater emphasis in clinics on supportive services. While the development of freestanding clinics has not resolved all problems of abortion service accessibility and should not totally replace hospital services, it has meant that safe, affordable abortion services have become increasingly available to most women in the United States.

TRENDS IN SERVICE PROVISION

Many freestanding abortion clinics were begun before 1973 in states that had liberalized their abortion laws, including some very large ones in California, Hawaii, New York, and Washington, D.C. In the early part of the decade, however, clinics represented a minority of providers. As shown in Table 1, in the first year of legal abortion throughout the country, 79 percent of all abortion service providers were hospital facilities which performed 52 percent of all abortions. These proportions decreased steadily each year, even between 1980 and 1982 when the number of abortions (1.5–1.6 million) and the abortion rate (30 per 1,000 women aged 15–44) remained quite stable. The percentage of all providers that were hospital facilities dropped to 48 percent by 1982 and, in that year, only 18 percent of all abortions occurred in hospitals.

As shown in Table 2, 27 percent of all abortion providers in 1982 were freestanding clinics; half of these were "abortion clinics," i.e., more than half their caseload came for abortions. Clinics, especially abortion clinics, are usually much

Table 1: Percent of Providers and Abortions in Hospitals

Year	Providers	Abortions
1973	79	52
1974	73	47
1975	68	40
1976	66	35
1977	62	30
1978	59	25
1979	56	23
1980	55	22
1981	52	20
1982	48	18

Table 2: Providers and Abortions by Type of Provider, 1982

Type	Providers	Abortions	Ab/Prov
Total	100%	100%	541
Hospitals	48	18	200
Clinics	27	77	1,544
Abortion	13	56	2,315
Other	14	21	832
MD Offices	25	5	104

larger than hospital facilities in that the average abortion clinic serves 11 times more patients than the average hospital and almost three times more than other types of clinics. The one percent of facilities serving 5,000 or more abortion patients annually accounts for 15 percent of all abortions. Most providers are much smaller. The 72 percent who serve fewer than 400 patients annually account for 11 percent of all abortions; 26 percent of all providers serve fewer than 30 patients per year. They account for less than one percent of all abortions in the U.S.

The change since legalization in the types of abortion providers in the U.S. has been the result of very little increase in the number of hospitals where abortions are provided--a 10 percent increase between 1973 and 1982--and large increases in the number of nonhospital providers. The number of freestanding clinics and private physician offices where abortions are provided was more than three times greater in 1982 than in 1973. These nonhospital facilities accounted for 90 percent of the net increase of 1,300 abortion service providers in the decade since legalization.

ACCESSIBILITY OF ABORTION SERVICE PROVIDERS

Hospitals that would be expected to provide abortion services (general, short-term, non-Roman Catholic hospitals) were only slightly more likely to do so in 1980 (27 percent) than in 1973 (24 percent) (see Table 3). The availability of abortion services in a hospital is determined by hospital policies about abortion services and by the willingness of physicians with privileges in a hospital to do abortions. Even

Table 3: Percent of General, Short-Term, Non-Catholic
Hospitals Providing Abortion Services

Year	Total	Metro	Nonmetro
1973	24	38	11
1980	27	42	13

at the present time, abortion services are not available in three out of four hospitals to which a woman might turn. Public hospitals on which many poor women must depend are less likely than private hospitals to offer abortion services (16 versus 32 percent, respectively). In addition, only 42 percent of obstetrician/gynecologists and 3 percent of general/family practitioners and general surgeons perform abortions (Orr and Forrest, 1985).

Women are likely to find abortion service providers more easily in metropolitan areas of the U.S. As Table 3 shows, metropolitan area hospitals are more than three times more likely to provide abortion services than are those in nonmetropolitan areas.

About 75 percent of U.S. women live in metropolitan areas, but 85 percent of all abortion providers are in metropolitan areas and 98 percent of all abortions occur there. Most women living in nonmetropolitan areas who need abortion services must travel to a metropolitan area to obtain them or forgo having an abortion. Indeed, since 1973, services have become more rather than less concentrated in metropolitan areas since most new providers chose to locate in cities.

Even now, 74 percent of nonmetropolitan area women live in counties with no abortion provider (see Table 4) and 96 percent live where there is no relatively large provider. In contrast, 14 percent of metropolitan area women live where there is no provider and 28 percent live in a county with no large facility. Overall, 28 percent of women in the U.S. live in a county with no abortion services provider. In 17 states, more than half of all women live where there is no provider. In response to such inequities in availability of abortion services, some 6 percent of women obtaining abortions in 1982 travelled to another state to do so. Abortion rates vary dramatically by state, from 10.9 per 1,000 among Kentucky residents to 44.9 per 1,000 women aged 15–19 in California (Henshaw et al., 1985). There is a high correlation between service availability and state abortion rates (Henshaw et al., 1982).

The percentage of abortions performed after the 12th week since the last menstrual period (LMP) has decreased from 14 percent in 1973 to 8.8 percent in 1981 (see Table 5). Many of these woman are having abortions beyond the first trimester of pregnancy because they have not recognized they were pregnant, a characteristic of many younger women who have not decided quickly on whether to obtain an abortion or have had difficulty locating a provider who will serve them or raising the money to pay for an abortion.

Finding a provider becomes increasingly difficult as a woman's gestation increases. Only 32 percent of all abortion service providers will serve a woman beyond 12 weeks LMP. Hospital providers are more likely to continue providing abortion services at later gestations. At 19 weeks LMP, when women diagnosed by amniocentesis to carry fetuses with genetic abnormalities would be seeking abortion services, 25 percent of all hospital providers but only 13 percent of abortion clinics would serve them. Only 5 percent of all providers still offer services at 21 weeks LMP.

Table 4: Percent of Women 15–44 in Counties
with No Abortion Provider, 1982

Total	28
Metro	14
Nonmetro	74

Table 5: Percent of Abortions at More Than 12 Weeks LMP

Year	More Than 12	More than 15	More than 20
1973	14.0	8.6	1.4
1981	8.8	4.0	0.9

As a result of the differences in the gestation at which services will be performed, hospital abortion service providers are especially important to women at later gestations. Abortions performed in hospital facilities are disproportionate at greater than 12 weeks LMP gestation (see Table 6). While 9 percent of all abortions are at 12 or more weeks gestation, 18 percent of those in hospital facilities are beyond the first trimester.

SAFETY BY TYPE OF PROVIDER

Mortality from abortion is now low in the United States. As seen in Figure 1 (from William Sappenfield of the CDC for AGI, 1986), at all gestations abortion mortality is less than maternal mortality although abortion mortality generally increases with gestation.

Three studies have looked at the comparative mortality risks of abortions performed in hospital and nonhospital settings. For both abortions at 12 weeks LMP or less (Grimes et al., 1978; Grimes et al., 1981) and those done by dilatation and evacuation at greater than 12 weeks LMP (Cates and Grimes, 1981), abortions in nonhospital settings showed lower mortality than those in hospitals. Some abortions are performed in hospital settings, however, because of certain health risks. When women who had health problems or who were undergoing additional surgery for sterilization were excluded from the comparison of those obtaining first trimester abortions, the mortality risks in hospital and nonhospital settings were equal.

Table 6: Percent of Abortions at More Than 12 Weeks LMP,
By Provider Type, 1982

Provider Type	Percent
Total	9
Hospital	18
Abortion Clinic	7
Other Clinic	6
MD Office	3

COMPARISON OF SERVICES BY TYPE OF PROVIDER

As shown in Table 7, 94 percent of all abortions in the U.S. in 1982 were outpatient procedures. This high proportion is due both to the large proportion of nonhospital procedures and to the fact that hospital abortions are increasingly becoming outpatient procedures. In 1982, only one-third of all hospital abortions were inpatient procedures, down from 45 percent in 1980. This trend has undoubtedly been influenced by the safety record of outpatient treatment and by the strong push in the U.S. to move medical treatment to outpatient settings in order to lessen the costs to both patients and insurers.

Abortion services in clinics cost about one-quarter of those performed in hospitals (Ory et al., 1982), in part because abortions at higher gestation and involving general rather than local anesthesia cost more. Still, at $200, the average total charge for a clinic abortion is less than just the average physician fee of $330 for a hospital procedure. Additional hospital charges average $445.

Surveys of clinic and hospital facilities (Lindheim, 1979; Henshaw, 1982; Landy and Lewit, 1982) have shown that not only are clinic abortion facilities more likely than hospitals to offer outpatient services and to cost less, but there are other factors that generally distinguish the different types of providers. In general, clinics are more likely than hospital facilities to provide abortion counseling, contraceptive counseling, contraceptive services, services to self-referred patients, and abortion services to minors on their own consent.

CONCLUSIONS

Since abortion services were legalized throughout the United States, the role of nonhospital clinics has increased steadily. This has been the result of very little change in the number of hospitals where abortions are performed while the number of nonhospital facilities more than tripled. Hospital facilities are still important, however, because abortion services are not very accessible in many areas of the country, because many poor women rely on public hospitals for medical care, and because hospitals provide a disproportionate amount of abortion care beyond the first trimester.

While hospitals remain important providers of abortion services in the United States, nonhospital clinics have been shown to be as safe as hospitals. Indeed, most hospitals have followed clinic experience by performing increasing proportions of abortions as outpatient procedures. Clinic abortions cost on average one-fourth of hospital procedures. In addition, clinics are often more accessible to women seeking abortion services and are more likely than hospitals to provide services like abortion and contraceptive counseling.

Table 7: Percent of Abortions as Inpatient Procedures
1980–1982

Year	Hosp. Abs.	All Abs.
1980	45	10
1981	38	8
1982	33	6

REFERENCES

Alan Guttmacher Institute (AGI). Induced Abortion, a World Review, 1985. 6th ed. AGI, New York, in press.

Cates, Jr., W., Grimes, D. A. Deaths from second trimester abortion by dilatation and evacuation: Causes, prevention, facilities. Obstetrics and Gynecology 58:401, 1981.

Grimes, D. A., Cates, Jr., W., Selik, R. M. Abortion facilities and the risk of death. Family Planning Perspectives 13:30, 1981.

Grimes, D. A., Cates, Jr., W., Tyler, Jr., C. W. Comparative risk of death from legally induced abortion in hospitals and nonhospital facilities. Obstetrics and Gynecology 51:323, 1978.

Henshaw, S. K. Freestanding abortion clinics: Services, structure, fees. Family Planning Perspectives 14:248, 1982.

Henshaw, S. K., Binkin, N. J., Blaine, E., Smith, J. C. A portrait of American women who obtain abortions. Family Planning Perspectives 17:90, 1985.

Henshaw, S. K., Forrest, J. D., Blaine, E. Abortion services in the United States, 1981 and 1982. Family Planning Perspectives 16:119, 1984.

Henshaw, S. K., Forrest, J. D., Sullivan, E., Tietze, C. Abortion services in the United States, 1979 and 1980. Family Planning Perspectives 14:5, 1982.

Landy, U., Lewit, S. Administrative, counseling and medical practices of abortion facilities. Family Planning Perspectives 14:257, 1982.

Lindheim, B. L. Services, policies and costs in U.S. abortion facilities. Family Planning Perspectives 11:283, 1979.

Orr, M. T., Forrest, J. D. The availability of reproductive health services from U.S. private physicians. Family Planning Perspectives 17:63, 1985.

Ory, H. W., Forrest, J. D., Lincoln, R. Making Choices: Evaluating the Health Risks and Benefits of Birth Control Methods. AGI, New York, 1983.

DELIVERY OF ABORTION CARE IN WESTERN EUROPE

Evert Ketting

Director of Research
STIMEZO Netherland
(National Abortion Federation of the Netherlands)
Zeist, The Netherlands

AN INTERNATIONAL COMPARATIVE STUDY ON ABORTION

In 1981 Stimezo Nederland* was asked by the German Ministry of Youth, Family, and Health to conduct a survey in which the actual working of abortion laws in Western Europe and the United States were to be evaluated. The question was whether these different laws produced differences in practice and whether such differences corresponded to the major aims of those laws. The background to this question was a notion that the new German abortion law, which was adopted in 1976, did not produce the intended effects. We undertook an extensive survey in which the abortion laws and practices of ten countries were studied comparatively. These countries were West Germany, Sweden, Denmark, the Netherlands, England, France, Austria, Switzerland, Italy, and the USA. After the survey was completed it turned out that the ministry, which by that time had changed from socialist to conservative, was not prepared to release the results. One and a half years later, and only after strong pressure from the media and the opposition parties, was permission for publication finally given. (Ketting and van Praag, 1985).

Some of the major outcomes of this study will be presented and discussed in this paper. They will focus on five questions:

1. Do restrictive abortion laws cause lower abortion rates, which is their main aim?

2. Does legal restriction to specified indications produce the intended effects?

3. Does restriction of abortion to the first trimester cause lower second trimester abortion rates?

4. What are the practical effects of permitting the performance of abortion only in general hospitals?

5. Which factors prevent or stimulate the much feared commercialization of abortion services?

---

* Stimezo Nederland: National Abortion Federation of the Netherlands, Koningsplein 38A, The Hague, The Netherlands.

LEGAL SITUATION IN WESTERN EUROPE

In 1967 England was the first country in the Western world to legalize abortion. This example was soon followed by most other Western countries. During the 1970s and early 1980s, the old restrictive abortion laws in Western Europe and in North America were, with a few exceptions, abolished or reformed. The development has resulted in an enormous diversity of legal situations. Table 1 presents an overview of this wide range of present-day legal situations.

This overview shows that abortion laws are most permissive in the Scandinavian countries and in Austria where abortion is allowed on the woman's request. In most Western European countries, however, a middle range solution has been adopted. These half-way liberalizations have essentially taken two forms. In the first, a specified indication is not required, but the forced counseling procedure is explicitly aimed at dissuading women from having an abortion and to adopt other solutions instead.

Table 1: Legal Abortion Situation in Western and
Southern Europe as of 1985

Country	Latest Major Legal Change	Most Permissive Indication	Until . . . Weeks since LMP	Forced Waiting Period
Group A: most permissive				
Sweden	1975	on request	18 weeks	none
(U.S.A.	1973	on request	± 24 weeks	none
Group B: highly permissive				
Denmark	1973	on request	12 weeks	none
Norway	1979	on request	12 weeks	none
Austria	1975	on request	± 15 weeks	none
Group C: moderately permissive				
France	1975	on request + dissuasion	12 weeks	7 days
Italy	1978	on request + dissuasion	13 weeks	7 days
Netherlands	1981	on request + dissuasion	viability	5 days
Group D: moderately restrictive				
England & Wales	1968	socio-medical	28 weeks	none
West Germany	1976	social + dissuasion	14 weeks	3 days
Switzerland	1942	socio-medical	undefined	none
Group E: highly restrictive				
Spain	1985	medical	12 weeks	none
Portugal	1984	medical	12 weeks	none
Belgium	19th century	medical	undefined	none
Group F: most restrictive				
Ireland	1983 referendum: constitutional prohibition of any abortion			

This is the case in France, Italy, and the Netherlands. In the second version abortion is only allowed on some specified legal ground, which has to be confirmed by a second doctor. Western Germany even has a combination of both solutions, allowing abortion only on medical or social (i.e., schwere Notlage) grounds and requiring counseling which is quite explicitly aimed at finding other solutions than abortion. In Spain, Portugal, and Belgium abortion is only permitted on strict medical indication and in Ireland abortion is prohibited in any case.

Strong political and social movements aiming at liberalizing the existing abortion laws are still present in 1985 in only two Western European countries, Belgium and Switzerland. The existing laws in both countries are generally felt to be most unsatisfactory.

It is important to note that the legal situations in these countries do not necessarily reflect actual practice. A restrictive law does not always mean that abortion is largely unavailable and a permissive legal situation does not always automatically lead to ample availability. For instance, it is much easier, cheaper, safer, and psychologically more acceptable to have an abortion in the Netherlands than to have one in Austria, although the law is more permissive in the latter country. Therefore, it is important to focus not only on legal aspects, but also on other conditions that shape the practice of abortion care. This is the intent of this paper.

LAW AND INCIDENCE OF ABORTION

Our survey had not shown a relationship between restrictiveness or permissiveness of the abortion law and the incidence of abortion. At the time of the survey, the Netherlands had one of the most liberal legal situations, and yet it had the lowest incidence of abortion. On the other hand, West Germany with its restrictive law showed an incidence comparable to that of Sweden and Denmark, where legal conditions were very permissive. According to the official statistics, the abortion incidence in West Germany is three times as low as is shown in Table 2, but the survey showed that these data are unreliable. Apparently, a major consequence of restrictive legislation is that many abortions are not reported, even when it is legally required, as is the case in West Germany. For instance, in West Berlin in 1981 only 2,700 abortions were reported to the Central Statistical Office, whereas 11,000 operations were known at the City Council to have taken place.

SPECIFIED INDICATIONS

In three of the countries studied--England, West Germany, and Switzerland --abortion is only permitted on certain specified legal grounds. The fact that these three countries do not have systematically lower abortion rates than countries where abortion is permitted on request indicates that these solutions do not produce the intended effects. In practice, indications do not work as selection criteria which differentiate between women with sufficient reasons to have an abortion and those women with insufficient reasons to get an abortion. In reality, indications fulfill the function of legal justifications of abortions which would be performed regardless of indications.

Table 2: Incidence of Abortion in Selected Western Countries (1980)

Country	Number of Abortions	Abortion Rate per 1,000 Women 15—44	Abortion Law
Netherlands	19,700	6.2	most permissive***
Switzerland	14,900	10.7	moderately restrictive
England & Wales	128,900	11.3	moderately restrictive
Italy*	222,400	18.8	moderately permissive
Sweden	34,800	20.5	most permissive
Denmark	23,300	21.3	highly permissive
France**	250,000	22.1	moderately permissive
W. Germany**	300,000	22.8	moderately restrictive
U.S.A.	1,553,900	29.6	most permissive

* Minimum estimate.
** Best estimate.
*** Tolerated practice.

This can be shown quite clearly when comparing these three countries. In England, a large majority of abortions are justified on medical grounds, in West Germany, about 80 percent are performed on social grounds,* and in Switzerland about 90 percent on psychiatric grounds. This simply means that the very same woman would get a medical indication in England, a social indication in West Germany, and a psychiatric indication in Switzerland. In Sweden or Denmark it would simply be called an abortion "on request."

Indications do not fulfill their intended function and cannot do so because they are usually too vague and are impossible to control. Since they only undermine the credibility of the law, it would be preferable to abolish them.

THE RESTRICTION TO THE FIRST TRIMESTER

Most abortion laws in Western Europe limit the performance of abortions during the second trimester of pregnancy to stricter criteria. However, when we look at practice, we have to conclude again that such rules hardly achieve the desired results. The percentage of second-trimester abortions in countries which restrict them is not systematically lower than in countries lacking such restrictions, although this sometimes appears to be the case when official statistics are compared. For instance, in our survey we found that the fairly reliable Danish statistics are not reliable. It turned out that a large number of second-trimester abortions are reported to be first-trimester ones. Since women with later gestations would otherwise have to go through a complicated procedure which could cause further delay.

* The percentage of abortions performed on social grounds has increased from only 44.9 percent, during the first half year after introduction of the new law in June 1976, to 83.3 percent in 1984 (Statistisches Bundesamt 1977; 1985).

THE PROHIBITION OF ABORTION IN PRIVATE PRACTICES AND SPECIALIZED ABORTION CLINICS

In the Scandinavian countries, France, Italy, and the southern states of West Germany abortion is only permitted to be performed in hospitals. In the Scandinavian countries this rule does not cause problems of access because abortion is largely accepted by the hospital administrations, the doctors, and other personnel. In Denmark, however, this rule has hampered the development toward outpatient abortion services which took place in most other countries with legalized abortion. Consequently, 85 percent of the procedures are inpatient.

In other countries this restriction has caused severe problems of access because, as is the case in the USA, many hospitals refuse to perform abortions. In France this problem has been solved by forcing hospitals to deliver abortion care, but in southern Germany the result has been abortion migration on a large scale. Many women from states like Bavaria and Baden-Wurttemberg travel to states where abortion outside hospitals is allowed or even go to Austria or the Netherlands.

THE COST OF ABORTION

The cost of abortion varies widely in Western Europe. In most countries the costs are covered by some kind of public health insurance program as is the case in the Scandinavian countries, England, West Germany, and Italy. In France it covers 75 percent of the cost and in the Netherlands the government only very recently decided to include abortion in the public health insurance program. Of the nine Western European countries studied, only Austrian and Swiss women have to pay for themselves. But reality again is different. First, coverage by a national health insurance program sometimes means that the incentive to lower the actual cost by delivering outpatient services is lacking. The result is that in West Germany, for example, the average hospital stay for an abortion is still about four days. Furthermore, coverage by a national health insurance program does not always mean that abortions are available free of charge for all women.

In England more than 50 percent of the women are forced to seek abortions in the private sector and to pay for them, because the National Health Service does not offer sufficient services. The West German women who are forced to travel abroad are sometimes facing heavy financial burdens, whereas in the restrictive regions of West Germany women are frequently charged with an additional, under-the-counter fee. In Austria and Switzerland fees for abortion services are usually extremely high, ranging from three to seven times the price which is normally paid in England or in the Netherlands.

In general our survey had indicated that the cost of abortion is particularly heightened by three factors, being (1) the restrictiveness of the law, (2) the taboo surrounding abortion, which causes a general lack of information about available services, and (3) coverage by a national insurance program.

CONCLUSIONS

The major conclusion of our survey has been that in practice, restrictive abortion legislation does not produce the intended effects. It does not lead to a decrease in the incidence of abortion. The so-called indications do not differentiate in practice between women with so-called sufficient or insufficent grounds. And finally, an extra barrier at the beginning of the second trimester does not cause lower second trimester abortion rates.

However, restrictive laws do produce negative effects, namely:

1. Unreliable data and therefore a false impression of reality.

2. Delay, causing more late abortions;

3. High prices for services;

4. Insufficient exchange of information on abortion care; and

5. Strengthening of the taboo surrounding abortion.

In short, the major consequence of restrictive legislation is bad practice.

REFERENCES

Ketting, E., van Praag, P. Schwangerschaftsabbruch, Gesetz und Praxis im internationalen Vergleich. DGVT-Verlag, Tubingen, 1985.

INDUCED ABORTION SERVICES IN ASIA

Rustom P. Soonawala

Honorary Medical Director
Family Planning Association of India
Professor--Obstetrics and Gynaecology
University of Bombay, India

INTRODUCTION

The termination of unwanted and unplanned pregnancy has been the practice of mankind ever since the beginning of civilization. Although it may not have been openly accepted, it has been widely practiced by all strata of society. Among the different countries of the world, abortion has been better accepted in Asian countries than others where undoubtedly there are reservations and restraints due to a strong influence of religion.

LEGAL PROFILE

On a broad basis, the legal profile of Asian countries can be grouped under three categories:

- Countries advocating a strict law whereby termination of pregnancy is not permitted even when it is hazardous to the health of the mother.

- Countries advocating a moderate law whereby termination is allowed if continuation of the pregnancy is hazardous to the mother's physical health.

  Most of these countries have allowed the practice of menstrual regulation since the procedure is performed before the pregnancy is diagnosed.

- Countries advocating a liberal law, whereby termination is allowed:

    - If the continuation of the pregnancy is hazardous to the mother's physical and mental health.

    - On socioeconomic grounds.

    - If pregnancy resulted due to failure of a contraceptive method.

TYPES OF ABORTION SERVICES AVAILABLE

A variety of abortion services are available and are grouped as:

187

1. Organized by the Government in their hospitals and primary health centers.

2. Organized by the Municipal health services in their hospitals and maternity homes.

3. Non Governmental Organizations (NGO)--Voluntary agencies involved in family welfare and health care through their clinics.

4. Private medical services in sophisticated, well-established hospitals or individual doctors' nursing homes or individual doctors' clinics.

5. Unauthorized illegal abortion services.

   These types of clinics are now few and scattered because good quality and safe services are available, but they still exist.

COST

The expense for undergoing termination of early pregnancy under 12 weeks would vary from nothing to about U.S.$100 equivalent in local currency.

The services are completely free in government and municipal centers so the patient need not pay anything.

In NGO clinics and charitable hospitals where abortion services are rendered on a not-for-profit basis the cost to the patient would be U.S.$5.00 to 7.00 equivalent in local currency.

In private hospitals and clinics the cost varies according to the individual patient ranging from the U.S. equivalent of $50 to $150.

It is important to understand that the establishment of good abortion services on a completely free basis is a cost-benefit measure. The expense incurred by the health authorities to hospitalize and treat women for complications due to illegal abortions performed under unhygienic conditions is exorbitant in comparison. In addition, the permanent damage in terms of high morbidity and frequent mortality associated with illegal abortion deserves serious consideration by the policy makers.

REPORTED FIGURES OF LEGAL ABORTION

In India the reported number of legal abortions is over a half million abortions per year. The impression is that another half million go unreported so that 1 million abortions per year would be the estimated number.

In the reported series the reasons listed are:

1. Danger to mother's life causing substantial risks   12.2%
2. Grave injury to physical health   17.8%
3. Grave injury to mental health   13.3%
4. Failure of contraception   49.4%
5. Rape (Unsolicited, Incest)   1.2%
6. Not available   6.1%

The age distribution is:

1.	Under 20 years	6.5%
2.	21 to 25 years	23.8%
3.	26 to 30 years	32.8%
4.	31 to 35 years	22.5%
5.	36 to 40 years	10.9%
6.	40 years & above	3.5%

The fear that with liberalization of the abortion law promiscuity would increase is without base. In this report 94 percent of women are over 20 years. Only 6 percent are younger than 20, the group which would include newly married or unmarried women requesting termination.

OBSERVATIONS

A woman caught with an unwanted pregnancy, anxious to terminate it, is in a vulnerable situation. If good, safe, and legal services for termination are not available, she will have to resort to so-called illegal abortion facing all the risks associated with it--high morbidity and mortality--and yet pay a fancy price.

All countries where abortion services are not freely available have illegal abortions performed in small or big ways. This setup encourages a clandestine practice causing unnecessary guilt and feelings of persecution in the doctor and the patient. There is no sane doctor who enjoys doing abortions just as there is no patient who enjoys undergoing an abortion. These are accidental, unwanted pregnancies which put the woman in the difficult situation of having to face all the criticism, while the male partner responsible for the pregnancy escapes without facing the consequences.

This is a time when sympathetic understanding and help are needed which cannot be extended if abortion services are unavailable.

It is a mistaken notion that abortions do not take place if the law prohibits them. They are either performed in a clandestine fashion or the individual is forced to travel to a neighboring country where services are readily and safely available.

CONCLUSION

Abortion as a method to control a quickly growing population is not an acceptable method. Abortion does, however, complement the contraceptive program of a country. The majority of women who undergo an abortion follow it by the use of a proper contraceptive method.

Termination of an unwanted pregnancy is a health care measure to reduce the maternal morbidity and mortality which is associated with illegal abortions.

COUNSELING AND ABORTION CARE

Uta Landy

Family Planning Consultant
San Francisco, California, U.S.A.

BACKGROUND

The shift from illegal to legal abortion in the United States represented a dramatic change for health care providers, the public, and individual women and their partners faced with unplanned pregnancy. Abortion, until then, bore the stigma of incompetent practitioners, and was equated with serious risks to women's health and even life. When women first began to seek legal abortions, they brought with them the taboos and fearful expectations which are part of illegal abortion. These were quickly transferred to the new, legal abortion clinics, their physicians, and staff and accusations of profiteering and abuse were soon made. Abortion providers needed to prove their professionalism and concern for the women they served. Women needed to be educated about safe and legal abortion and needed to be reassured. It was a common notion that women could not make the abortion decision alone, that they needed professional help. The establishment of counseling as an integral part of the abortion service served these purposes. Providing information, support, and guidance by a professional counselor in conjunction with a medical service was and is an exemplary practice. Counseling has, after more than a decade of legal abortion, come to be perceived as beneficial to patients and providers.

CURRENT PRACTICE OF COUNSELING IN THE UNITED STATES

Aborting counseling as it is currently practiced in the United States relies on three assumptions:

1. That the woman is entitled to information about the abortion and its risks and alternatives;

2. That prevention, i.e., contraception, is essential; and

3. That the choice to terminate or not terminate a pregnancy must be the woman's.

According to standards developed by the National Abortion Federation in the U.S.A., counseling should:

1. Provide the opportunity to explore the woman's feelings about the pregnancy and her options.

2. Assist in decision-making if needed.

3. Ensure informed consent.

4. Prepare the woman for surgery to facilitate her safety and comfort.

5. Assist the woman in choosing a method of contraception (NAF, 1984).

When abortions were first legalized, help with decision-making was considered the most essential aspect of counseling. More than a decade later, most women have enough access to information about their options that they do not require help in making a decision by the time they have made an appointment at an abortion clinic. Some women still seek assistance or support with their decision, sometimes openly, but often in a less direct and obvious way. An experienced counselor can recognize hostile, withdrawn, or nonchalant behavior as an expression of conflict and can offer these women special time and assistance in clarifying feelings and reviewing options in an accepting and nonjudgmental atmosphere (Landy, 1986).

Informed consent for abortion, as for any medical procedure, is to ensure that the patient makes a decision and agrees to the abortion with a full understanding of her options and the medical risks involved. Questions about the woman's ability to give informed consent only arise if she is retarded, severely emotionally disturbed, or very young. In such cases, a responsible adult, usually a relative of the woman, is consulted. The involvement of another adult may be prescribed by law or left to the judgment of the counselor or physician.

Once the woman has decided to terminate her pregnancy she must be given practical information about appointment times and schedules, physical and laboratory examinations, the method of abortion, and the feelings and sensations which she can expect to experience. The better the woman is prepared and informed, the more relaxed and less fearful she will be. Proper education is essential in reducing anxiety and fear associated with any medical procedure.

CONTRACEPTIVE COUNSELING

The goal of contraceptive counseling is to help the woman avoid future unplanned pregnancies. In the context of an abortion service, the practice of preventive medicine requires a discussion of contraceptive methods and their risks and benefits. To help her use contraception successfully, it may also be necessary to explore the woman's feelings about her sexuality, her relationship, and her feelings toward various birth control methods. Pre-abortion counseling may be the first opportunity for a woman to evaluate her contraceptive practices and to gain sufficient information and motivation for a new start.

Counselors must be aware of and recognize their personal bias toward a particular contraceptive method and refrain from directing the woman toward or away from the method of their own personal choice or bias (Beresford, 1979). Studies have shown that a woman's contraceptive success depends on her commitment and a variety of psychosocial factors (Furstenberg, 1976; Luker, 1975; Sachdev, 1985). Instead of simply recounting the available birth control methods and their effectiveness in a group setting, as is commonly done in United States clinics, contraceptive counseling is best done in a private setting and should be tailored to the woman's knowledge and individual needs.

EMOTIONAL SUPPORT

When a woman must decide how to respond to an unplanned pregnancy, she is forced to evaluate her life, her relationship with her family, her husband or her sexual partner, and her role as a woman in society. Whatever decision she reaches, she carries the responsibility and it is she who suffers the physical and emotional consequences of childbirth or an abortion. Within each component of abortion counseling--decision-making guidance, informed consent, education, and contraceptive counseling--the objective must be emotional support and comforting. Emotional support can be expressed by:

1. Being empathetic.

2. Establishing rapport, i.e., being genuinely interested in the patient and her concerns.

3. Listening well by maintaining eye contact, nodding.

4. Allowing the woman to express her feelings.

5. Avoiding negative judgments about the woman's life or feelings.

Many women who make the decision to terminate a pregnancy experience a mixture of happy and sad feelings ranging from a sense of relief to sadness and mourning over a potential child. Women who would like to have a child but feel forced to postpone parenthood because of economic, health, or relationship circumstances are especially likely to experience grieving and a sense of loss. Such feelings should be distinguished from genuine feelings of confusion and ambivalence which may not be resolved in the course of a brief counseling session but warrant referral for professional psychological help.

QUALIFICATIONS OF COUNSELORS

The abortion clinics in the U.S.A. employ counselors with a variety of educational and professional backgrounds. A college or graduate degree in the social sciences might be helpful, but personal attributes are considered to be of greatest importance (Hern, 1985; Landy, 1986). Personal warmth, a positive outlook on life, empathy and caring, self-discipline, a cooperative attitude, comfort with her own and others' sexuality, and willingness to learn are mentioned as desirable counselor traits (NAF, 1984; Hern, 1985).

Training for counselors generally takes place in the clinic itself and is conducted by senior counselors, administrators or physicians. Counselors are occasionally offered the opportunity for training through professional seminars conducted by the National Abortion Federation, Planned Parenthood Federation of America or one of its affiliates, or a training institute specializing in family planning. According to the Standards of the National Abortion Federation (1984), initial training of counselors must include:

1. Sexual and reproductive health.

2. Abortion technology.

3. Contraceptive technology.

4. Short-term counseling skills.

5. Community resources and referrals.

6. Informed consent.

7. Agency policies and procedures.

GROUP VERSUS INDIVIDUAL COUNSELING

Group and individual counseling offer different advantages and disadvantages. The group setting can provide potential sources of support because members can share their feelings, reassure each other, and develop a sense of comradery which can continue through the entire time spent at the clinic (Landy and Lewit, 1982; Sachdev, 1985). Individual counseling, on the other hand, offers a patient the privacy to discuss personal concerns and ask questions which she may feel too shy or embarrassed to ask in a group setting. Studies conducted shortly after the legalization of abortion confirmed the benefits of group counseling (Burnell et al., 1972; Bracken et al., 1973). Use of individual or group counseling by a particular clinic depends on the views of the head counselor, the administrator, or physician and such practical aspects as available space, patient flow, and the number of counselors. A survey of the member clinics of NAF (which perform about half of all abortions in the U.S.A.) showed that 39 percent of the clinics offer group counseling sometimes or never, 35 percent use individual counseling sometimes or never, 27 percent offer individual counseling exclusively, and 28 percent provide both group and individual counseling always or usually (Landy and Lewit, 1982).

FORMAT AND TIMING OF COUNSELING

While the content of counseling generally adheres to those areas outlined by the Standards, the format and timing of counseling can vary from clinic to clinic. Contraceptive counseling, for example, may consist of audiovisual presentations describing the available methods, their use, risks, and benefits, followed by personal consultation with the counselor.

Timing of contraceptive counseling can vary as well. It may be included in the initial counseling session, or it may be offered after the abortion, i.e., during recovery, or at the time of the follow-up visit. Some counselors believe that a patient is less receptive to information before the abortion when she is preoccupied with anticipating the operation. In this case, contraceptive counseling is postponed until after the procedure. If the patient is likely to return to the clinic for a follow-up visit (a regular patient at the clinic, for example), contraceptive counseling may even be postponed until then. When patients must travel to the clinic or have their own physician or medical facility elsewhere, contraceptive counseling should take place at the time of the abortion. It should never be assumed that someone else will provide it.

The responsibilities of the counselor also vary from clinic to clinic. In some facilities, the counselor helps the patient complete registration and consent forms, performs the counseling, prepares the woman for surgery, stays with the woman during the abortion to comfort her, and assists her during recovery. In other clinics, one counselor performs the counseling while another counselor accompanies the woman through the abortion and recovery. Some counselors have contact with the patient only once, during the actual counseling session, while other staff, usually a nurse, see the woman through the abortion and recovery. Whether a counselor stays with the woman during the abortion may also depend on the type of anesthesia used. When local anesthesia is used a counselor often stays with the woman in the operating room, holds her hand, speaks with her, explains the progession of the operation to her, and helps her to stay calm and relaxed. Counseling is often offered to the woman's partner or relative. Eighty-seven percent of the NAF clinics made such counseling available.

It is difficult to determine the effectiveness of counseling. Studies to this effect are sparse and inconclusive (Sachdev, 1985), but more than a decade of legal abortion in the U.S. has convinced those involved in the provision of abortion services that counseling, albeit modified since the first years after legalization, is a necessary component of abortion care and is perceived as helpful by the physician performing the abortion and the woman having the abortion (Hern, 1984).

The practice of abortion counseling has been widely accepted in the U.S. and in Europe and, as other chapters of this volume indicate, this approach is beginning to find accpetance in the developing world as well. Women need to be educated about reproduction and they need emotional support in their difficult reproductive roles. These needs transcend culture, economics, and politics. Content and form of that support is influenced by a number of factors, such as:

1. The role of women in society.

2. Religious sanctions.

3. Fear of pain, injury, and death.

4. Public acceptance of family planning and abortion.

Some cultures specify appropriate roles for women--that they marry at a certain age and refrain from sexual activity prior to marriage, that they have a minimum number of children, an expectation which may vary between rural and urban women, or in population-conscious countries such as China, a maximum number of children, that childbearing should be postponed even after marriage until the couple is economically well established, an expectation which is influenced by social status and class. In a society such as the United States, the messages are ambivalent, especially for teenagers. The teenager is expected to be "sexy" and is constantly titillated by sexual innuendos through the mass media, but the messages about sexual activity are unclear. Such lack of clarity is bound to cause conflict for the teenager about sexuality, the use of contraception, and resolution of an unintended pregnancy.

However clear or mixed the cultural or societal expectations, the counselor's effectiveness is enhanced by knowing about them and acknowledging them with and for the woman. A cross-cultural perspective can enhance and clarify the understanding of one's own social and political expectations as other chapters of this book demonstrate.

An international comparison of religious attitudes toward fertility control can also help counselors understand women's feelings and conflicts regarding contraception and abortion. Religious influences vary in different societies and may affect fertility practice or attitude. Despite staunch opposition by the Catholic Church, abortions are legal in Italy, the seat of the Church, while the Church's influence in South America has seriously hampered any efforts to legalize abortion there. The degree of a woman's religiosity and the extent to which she separates religion from the pragmatic aspects of her life will determine the extent to which religion will influence her decisions and feelings about fertility control.

Fear of pain, injury, and death in anticipation of surgery are universal, but cultures vary in the ways in which people cope with those fears. Some cultures promote stoicism toward pain and positive attitudes about death. A woman's expectation of any medical procedure, including her cultural associations with blood, pain, and surgical instruments and her tolerance of pain will influence the degree of anxiety and tension with which she anticipates and tolerates the operation.

A woman's feelings about contraception and abortion are also influenced by the degree of public acceptance of fertility control. If abortion is illegal, it is often dangerous and warrants a negative perception. But even when abortion and contraception are legal and generally available, they may not have an official stamp of approval either by government or society at large. Negative political and public attitudes prevent broad-based education about reproduction and fertility control through schools, the media, and other social institutions. Instead, women are more likely to feel guilt and anxiety and lack the necessary information to make rational decisions about their fertility.

In order to respond sensitively to the woman's needs for information and support during abortion and contraceptive counseling, the social climate must be considered. Regardless of the woman's role in society, religious influences, fears about pain and injury, and the social acceptance of contraception or abortion, all women need and deserve accurate information, understanding, and empathy about their family planning decisions just as they do with other medical decisions affecting their lives and health.

REFERENCES

Beresford, T. Abortion counseling. In G. I. Zatuchni, J. J. Sciarra, J. J. Speidel, eds., Pregnancy Termination. Harper & Row, Hagerstown, Maryland, 1979.

Bracken, M. B., Grossman, G., Hachamovitch, M., et al. Abortion counseling: An experimental study of three techniques. Americal Journal of Obstetrics and Gynecology 117:10, 1973.

Burnell, E. M., Sworsky, W. A., Harrington, R. L. Post-abortion group therapy. American Journal of Psychiatry 129(2):220, 1972.

Furstenberg, F. F. Unplanned Parenthood. The Free Press, New York, 1976.

Hern, W. M. Abortion Practice. J. B. Lippincott Co., Philadelphia, 1984.

Landy, U. Abortion counselling--A new component of medical care. In J. J. La Ferla, ed., Clinics in Obstetrics and Gynecology, 13,1. W. B. Saunders Co., London, 1986.

Landy, U., Lewit, S. Administrative, counseling, and medical practices of National Abortion Federation facilities. Family Planning Perspectives 14:5, 1982.

Luker, K. Taking Chances: The Decision Not to Contracept. University of California Press, Berkeley, 1975.

National Abortion Federation. Standards for Quality Care. Washington, D.C., 1984.

Sachdev, P. Counseling single abortion patients: A research overview and practice implications. In P. Sachdev, ed., Perspectives on Abortion. The Scarecrow Press, Metuchen, New Jersey, 1985.

CONTRACEPTION AFTER PREGNANCY TERMINATION

Allan Rosenfield

Dean, School of Public Health
Director, Center For Population and Family Health
Columbia University
New York, U.S.A.

INTRODUCTION

Very simply put, contraceptive counseling and services are an essential component of any abortion service program. In fact, it is fair to say that contraception should be an integral part of all reproductive health care, particularly post-abortion and postpartum. It is unfortunately true that the general obstetrics and gynecology community, over the years, has given inadequate attention to this area, particularly for low-income clinic patients. The situation has been somewhat better in private practice but even here it is often the woman who initiates the discussion rather than the physician offering contraceptive counseling as an integral part of the health care process.

Currently in the United States most, but not all, abortion clinics provide contraceptive counseling and service, but the literature is spotty and no effective national reporting system exists to assist us in this process. Internationally, there is even less information. Data from the United States, however, are promising concerning post-abortion contraceptive use. The pregnancy rate among sexually active adolescents has decreased from 6 percent since abortion was legalized in 1973 and contraceptive use at last intercourse increased by 39 percent between 1971 and 1979 (AGI, 1981).

In the early 1970s the pioneering PRETERM Clinic in Washington, D.C., offered contraceptive counseling and services routinely as a part of their program and as a component of the abortion fee. The concept of an all-inclusive fee including contraception is a model for almost all abortion services (Margolis et al., 1974). At PRETERM 400 women were studied. Ninety percent accepted contraception post-abortion, and, in a follow-up 6 months later in which 75 percent of all original clients were contacted by telephone at home, 90 percent of those who had accepted contraception were still using a method, an unusually high figure. During the year of the study, PRETERM provided care for 20,000 women, most of whom accepted contraception. At least at this clinic most women did not choose to continue to be exposed to the risk of repeat abortions.

In the United States, two sociologists, Kantner and Zelnick, conducted a landmark longitudinal study on teenage sexuality, pregnancy and contraceptive practice, which included surveys of teenagers in 1971, 1976, and 1979 (Zelnick and Kantner, 1980). One of their findings demonstrated that teenagers whose first pregnancy ended in an abortion were half as likely to become pregnant in one year as compared to those who delivered a live birth.

In 1981, Westoff and his colleagues at Princeton published a report on a 15-clinic study in Illinois in which there was a 4,133 patient sample (Westoff et al., 1981). At conception, 58 percent had been using no method, a rate that rose to 73 percent for young women under the age of 20. Thirteen percent used the pill, 2 percent the IUD, and 6 percent the condom. After the abortion, their data suggested that only 3 percent were not planning to use a method, including only 6 percent among adolescents, with 61 percent using or planning to use the pill (79 percent for women under the age of 20), 11 percent the IUD, and 3 percent the condom. In addition, 11 percent of women over the age of 20 underwent a sterilization procedure.

In this study it was estimated that 70 percent of abortions in the United States could be averted if all women at risk used the pill or the IUD. The percentage is not higher because 25 percent of adolescents and almost 50 percent of those over the age of 20 years were using contraception when they became pregnant. Thus, even with contraceptive use, 10 percent of adolescent contraceptive users and 14 percent of adult users will become pregnant each year, leading to some 450,000 abortions per year, a drop from the current level of about 1.6 million abortions annually. The contraceptive failure points up problems with our current contraceptive methods, demonstrating clearly the urgent need for continued and expanded contraceptive research.

METHODS OF CONTRACEPTION POST-ABORTION

It has been demonstrated that in those women undergoing a first trimester suction currettage procedure, with no sign of pelvic inflammatory disease, the post-abortion insertion of an IUD does not increase early complications (Rosenfield and Castadot, 1974). For women in stable relationships, post-abortal insertion of an IUD is an appropriate alternative to be offered. However, sexually active teenagers who usually are in more unstable relationships are at a higher risk of pelvic inflammatory disease and thus post-abortal insertion of IUD is not recommended.

IUDs can probably also be inserted immediately post-abortion after second-trimester D&E procedures although there are no specific data available in this regard. Indirect evidence exists, however, from extensive experience, particularly in Asia. During the 1960s and 1970s the Population Council conducted a Postpartum Program in which well over 100,000 women received an IUD within 2 or 3 days after delivery (Rosenfield and Castadot, 1974). Successful insertion and a low expulsion rate depends on insertion of the IUD high into the fundus. If the IUD is inserted in the normal way, however, it will usually end up in the lower uterine segment and be expelled.

Perhaps the most widely used post-abortal method is the pill, which should be started within the first few days following the abortion since it is likely that the woman will ovulate in the first cycle post-abortion. There are no data to suggest that current methods of pregnancy termination lead to an increased incidence of thromboembolic phenomenon, and thus there is no reason to delay the initiation of hormonal contraception. For those women who are at risk of cardiovascular complications for other reasons, initiation of pill use should be delayed and barrier methods recommended instead.

Although the drug is not currently available for contraceptive use in the United States, medroxyprogesterone acetate (DMPA or Depo-provera) would be a most appropriate method for use post-abortion. Despite the USFDA decision not to approve this drug, it has been recommended as appropriate for contraceptive use by toxicology review committees of the World Health Organization, by the American College of Obstetricians and Gynecologists, by the Medical Advisory Panel of the International Planned Parenthood Federation, and the drug regulatory agencies in many other countries, including, most recently, Sweden, West Germany, Great Britain, and Canada (Rosenfield and Maine, 1980). In some of these countries the approval is for use when other methods are not available, while in Canada it is for general use. The drug has been well accepted where it has been used.

A new method, NORPLANT, consists of a series of silastic rods impregnated with levonorgesterol which is implanted subdermally in the upper arm. NORPLANT holds great promises as a general and post-abortion contraceptive method (Sivin et al., 1982). It has been approved for use in Finland, the country of manufacture, Sweden, and other countries in the developing world. USFDA approval is expected within the next year or two.

Sterilization as a post-abortal procedure is a more complex issue. It has been proven safe to perform a sterilization procedure postabortion, but the potential for coercion, particularly among low-income populations, is great. Therefore, although there is disagreement on this issue, it is questionable whether an informed consent can be obtained at the time of the abortion.

ABORTION, CONTRACEPTION, AND THE ADOLESCENT

Ten percent of the world's population are in the 15—19 age group, which amounts to about 500 million adolescents, 85 percent of whom live in the developing world. As an example of the rapid rate of increase, the adolescent population in Latin America will double over the next 35 years and will increase by three times in Africa during the same period of time. The birthrate among adolescents in the United States is approximately 50 per 1,000, with the majority occurring among unmarried teenagers. In Bangladesh, on the other hand, the rate is five times higher (250 per 1,000), almost all occurring among married teenagers, many of whom were married at a very young age.

There is an increasing rate of sexual activity among unmarried teenagers worldwide, particularly in urban areas. In the developing world, much of teenage sexual activity takes place within marriage in traditional rural societies. But with the breakdown of family and cultural ties in the urban slums of many of the developing world cities, teenage sexual activity is increasing with an increase in out-of-wedlock pregnancy, illegal abortion, and childbirth. There is a need for better data on adolescents in developing countries, particularly in regard to illegal abortion. For those who do become pregnant and do submit to an abortion, whether legal or illegal, contraceptive counseling and services should be offered wherever possible. This is clearly a problem in the case of illegal abortion, but certainly for those young women who are hospitalized with complications of a septic abortion, contraceptive counseling, services, and follow-up are essential components of the patient's overall care.

In Latin America, it is estimated that illegal abortions among both adolescent and adult women account for more maternal deaths than any other single cause (Rosenfield and Maine, 1985). The world, by and large, has ignored the problem of illegal abortion, which may kill as many as 100,000 to 200,000 women each year. Overall, WHO estimates that maternal mortality rates in the developing world are from 10 to 100 times those in the West, with more than 500,000 women dying each year of pregnancy-related complications (including illegal abortion), most of which are preventable with existing technology. This constitutes one of the world's most neglected health tragedies. The time has come to mount a major and urgent campaign to decrease preventable maternal deaths from high-parity and out-of-wedlock pregnancies. Illegal abortion is a particular tragedy and the world's health community must react with appropriate preventive contraceptive and abortion services. For those women undergoing an abortion, contraception must be an integral component of care.

REFERENCES

Alan Guttmacher Institute. Teenage pregnancy: The problem that hasn't gone away. In Factbook on Teenage Pregnancy. The Alan Guttmacher Institute, New York, 1981.

Margolis, A., Rindfuss, R., Coghlan, P., et al. Contraception after abortion. Family Planning Perspectives 6:56, 1974.

Rosenfield, A., Castadot, R. G. Early postpartum and immediate post-abortion Intrauterine contraceptive device insertion. American Journal of Obstetrics and Gynecology 118(8):1104, 1974.

Rosenfield, A., Maine, D. Maternal mortality--A neglected tragedy. Where is the M in MCH? The Lancet, p. 83, July 1985.

Rosenfield, A., Maine, D., Rochat, R., et al. The Food and Drug Administration and medroxyprogesterone acetate. What are the issues? Journal of the American Medical Association 249(21):2922, June 3, 1983.

Sivin, I., Diaz, S., Holmes, P., et al. A four-year clinical study of NORPLANT implants. Studies in Family Planning 13:258, 1982.

Westoff, C. F., Delung, J. S., Goldman, N., Forrest, J. D. Abortions preventable by contraceptive practice. Family Planning Perspectives 13:204, 1981.

Zelnick, M., Kantner, J. F. Sexual activity, contraceptive use and pregnancy among metropolitan area teenagers, 1971–1979. Family Planning Perspectives 12:230, 1980.

THE MAGNITUDE OF MATERNAL MORTALITY:

DEFINITIONS AND METHODS OF MEASUREMENT

Roger W. Rochat

Professor
Department of Community Health
Emory University School of Medicine
and
Medical Epidemiologist
Office of the Director
Centers for Disease Control
Atlanta, Georgia, U.S.A.

INTRODUCTION

Over 200 million women become pregnant each year and 130 million bear children. Each year nearly 500,000 women die as a result of complications of pregnancy or childbearing. Ninety-nine percent of these deaths would be prevented if the lowest mortality rates in developed countries were achieved worldwide. Moreover, all regions of the World Health Organization (WHO) give high priority to lowering maternal mortality to achieve 'Health for All' by the year 2000. Even in developed countries with low maternal mortality, such as the United States, an estimated 50 percent or more of maternal deaths are preventable--and lowering the rate to five per 100,000 live births is among the United States' stated public health priorities.

How do we know how many die? The lack of any data in many countries about maternal mortality and fatalistic attitudes toward pregancy and childbearing have obscured the importance and preventability of this health problem.

The World Health Organization's Division of Family Health Services has contributed a landmark report on maternal mortality rates from different regions and countries of the world and is preparing a monograph on the subject which will aid all of us in our efforts to improve maternal health (World Health Organization, 1985).

In this paper we compare several definitions of maternal mortality, describe methods of data collection, briefly summarize the WHO data and describe and present three different approaches to studying maternal mortality in developing areas: Taiwan, Zambia, and Bangladesh.

DEFINITIONS

Three definitions of maternal death and recommended definitions of maternal mortality rates are shown in Table 1-1. There are two points of controversy. Should maternal deaths include only those deaths occurring within 42 days after

201

Table 1-1: Definition of Maternal Death

MATERNAL DEATH

* Maternal death is the death of a woman known to be pregnant or within 42 days of delivery or termination of pregnancy, irrespective of the duration of or site of the pregnancy. (WHO, 1984)

* Maternal death is the death of any woman, from any cause, while pregnant or within 42 days of termination of pregnancy, irrespective of the duration and the site of pregnancy. (ACOG, 1974)--(Note the American Medical Association uses a 90-day interval.)

* Maternal death is the death of a woman from any cause related to or aggravated by pregnancy or its management (regardless of duration or site of pregnancy), but not from accidental or incidental causes. (ACOG, 1985; Cefalo, 1985)

pregnancy termination or should the time frame be 90 days or one year? Second, should it include or exclude nonmaternal deaths? The American College of Obstetricians and Gynecologists (ACOG) recommends no time limit for comparisons within the United States (American College of Obstetricians and Gynecologists, 1985); the World Health Organization recommends a 42-day limit for international comparisons (World Health Organization, 1977). Most investigators collect data including nonmaternal deaths but exclude nonmaternal deaths in computing maternal mortality rates, and official definitions reflect this approach.

The primary purpose of a definition used internationally is to compare trends and mortality rates among countries where data vary substantially in quality. The current WHO definition of a maternal death appears to serve this purpose well. However, the use of a 42-day interval may serve primarily to exclude pregnancy-related deaths outside the 42-day interval, rather than improving the completeness of reporting of deaths within the 42-day interval.

Definitions used by different state health departments and local maternal mortality committees in the United States vary widely; the proposed changes in ACOG's definition reflect a broader inclusion temporarily but a greater restriction in possible causal relations (Cefalo, 1985). For some obstetricians the additional clinical distinction between direct, indirect, and nonmaternal deaths helps identify those causes of death most likely preventable by clinicians (Table 1-2). However, as clinical interventions become increasingly successful, nonmaternal causes may represent the larger portions of the public health problem.

Whether the denominator is 1,000, 10,000, or 100,000 usually depends on the level of maternal mortality. WHO has in the past recommended 10,000, but 100,000 is widely used. For comparison, live births are most commonly used as the denominator, but live and stillbirths, or number of maternities, or pregnancies, are also used. The latter is appropriate for computing relative risks of dying from pregnancy. Each of these definitions is a ratio and not a true rate, which would require including all pregnant women in the denominator.

An epidemiologic approach to studying maternal mortality would require identification of all deaths among women of reproductive age and determination of those which are temporarily associated with pregnancy and its sequelae and then determination of those causes of death occurring significantly more frequently among pregnant than nonpregnant women. Presumably most clinically defined direct and indirect causes would be epidemiologically attributable to pregnancy.

Table 1-2: Clinical Classification of Maternal Deaths

Direct Maternal Death: an obstetric death resulting from obstetric complications of the pregnancy state, labor, or puerperium and from interventions, omissions, incorrect treatment, or chain of events resulting from any of these complications.

Indirect Maternal Death: An obstetric death resulting from previously existing disease, or disease that developed during pregnancy, labor, or the puerperium. It is not due to direct obstetric causes, although the physiologic effects of pregnancy were partially responsible for the death.

Nonmaternal Death: An obstetric death resulting from accidental (e.g., gunshot wounds, auto accidents) or incidental (e.g., concurrent malignancy) causes not related to the pregnancy or its management

---

For example, obstetrical hemorrhage, puerperal infection, and hypertensive cerebrovascular accidents also occur in the absence of pregnancy. Indirect causes such as hepatitis and malaria have higher death-to-case rates for pregnant than nonpregnant women.

Of even greater interest might be the presumed nonmaternal deaths temporarily associated with pregnancy. Are violent deaths from personal injury--homicide, suicide, and trauma from vehicular accidents--more or less common among pregnant than nonpregnant women?

To my knowledge, no systematic epidemiologic studies have ever been conducted on pregnancy as a risk factor for deaths from intentional or unintentional injury. Consider the following examples. First, fatalities from vehicular accidents have been associated with the rapid transport of women in labor to the hospital. Second, in May 1985 a nationally publicized homicide occurred in New Jersey because a boy did not want his pregnant girlfriend to obtain an abortion. He burned her house down. Five others died in the same fire. (Atlanta Journal, 1985).

A third example might be suicide after abortion. The U.S. Centers for Disease Control reports it identifies over 90 percent of deaths during or shortly after abortion (Cates, 1978). Between 1972 and 1981 only three suicides were reported after 9.9 million abortions, a rate of .03 per million abortions. Assuming women are at risk for suicide associated with abortion for three months after abortion, the secular age- and sex-adjusted suicide rates would imply that 124 suicides should have occurred shortly after abortion. This implies either that suicide after abortion is markedly underreported to CDC, or that pregnancy terminated by abortion may protect a woman from suicide. These hypotheses need evaluation.

Only through epidemiologic studies comparing mortality risks for pregnant and nonpregnant women can we learn the nonreproduction risks and benefits of pregnancy to the health of women. Until they have been conducted, we would recommend including nonmaternal deaths in the broad definition of maternal death and using the tools of epidemiology to determine the contribution of the pregnancy to dying.

The temporal relationship of a woman's death to pregnancy and its outcome is crucial in assessing and attributing risk, but this temporal relationship cannot be determined by data on death certificates. The death certificate has no place to report the interval since last pregnancy ended. The importance of temporal relationships is demonstrated in three ways.

1. The Ninth International Classification of Disease (ICD) sequences its seven major subcategories of maternal death according to the temporal cause of the pregnancy (Table 2).

2. For induced abortion the death-to-case rate rises with increasing duration of pregnancy (Figure 1). In the United States the absolute risk of dying after abortion and the relative risk of mortality at later gestations declined during the 1970s.

3. Different definitions of maternal deaths include intervals of 42, 60, 90, and 365 days or longer after the pregnancy is completed. Special studies linking birth certificates to deaths of women of reproductive years demonstrate that the number of maternal deaths occurring more than 42 days after completion of pregnancy may represent 16 percent or more of the pregnancy-related deaths (Rubin, 1981).

SOURCES OF DATA

In developing countries, data on maternal deaths are usually obtained through hospital data or surveillance such as vital registration which certify vital events (Table 3). Hospital data on maternal deaths may have the most medically correct cause of death information, but hospitals selectively underreport selected causes, such as deaths from abortion and ectopic pregnancy, and deaths of poorer and rural women. In some settings, moribund women are discharged from the hospital to die at home because it costs the family more to transport a dead person home for burial than a moribund person home to die.

Vital statistics systems report vital events routinely without special effort to ensure completeness of reporting or accuracy of cause of death data. The most common examples are death certificates signed by physicians or registration of vital events by household. Church burial information has been used to estimate maternal mortality by computing excess female deaths for adults aged 15−44. Reports of deaths in newspapers have been used in Japan to detect suicides associated with pregnancy. Reports by hospitals and health workers may facilitate the correct classification of deaths due to maternal causes, and identify those maternal deaths recognized by health workers.

The best information is obtained from multiple sources in a defined population. Complete ascertainment of maternal deaths requires either (1) careful investigation of causes of deaths among all women of reproductive age or those identified as occurring during the postpartum interval, (2) prospective surveillance of pregnant women and pregnancy outcomes, or (3) household surveys. The last two options

Table 2: Major Subcategories for Classifying Deaths Due to Complications of Pregnancy, Childbirth, and the Puerperium

ICD CODE

630–633	Ectopic and Molar Pregnancy (excludes choriocarcinoma)
634–639	Other Pregnancy with Abortive Outcome
640–649	Complications Mainly Related to Pregnancy
650–659	Normal Delivery, and Other Indications for Care in Pregnancy, Labor, and Delivery
660–669	Complications Occurring Mainly in the Course of Labor and Delivery
670–676	Complications of the Puerperium

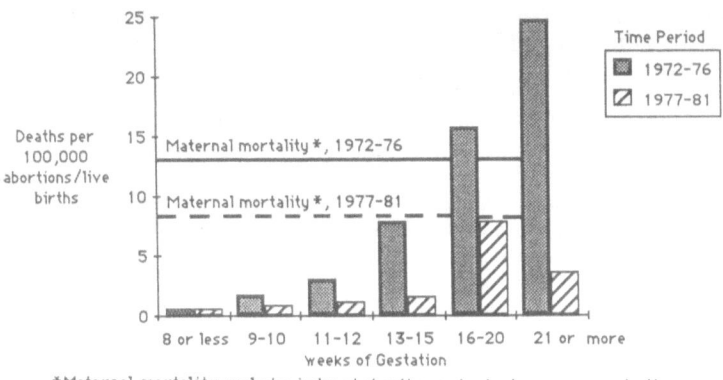

Fig. 1. Deaths per 100,000 Legal Abortions by Weeks of
Gestation and Maternal Mortality per 100,000 Live Births,
United States, 1972-76 and 1977-81.

Table 3: Methods for Detecting Maternal Deaths

---

1. Surveillance of defined population

    a.   Vital Statistics

         · Routine Death Certificate reports
         · Birth-Death Linked Records
         · Investigate reported deaths of women 12–49

    b.   Community studies

         · Identify all deaths of women 12–49; investigate causes
         · Household probability survey
         · Identify all pregnant women; observe until 6 or more weeks after
           pregnancy ends

    c.   Confidential inquiries

         · Vital statistics + investigate maternal death reports
         · Multiple source reports + investigate maternal deaths

2. Surveillance when at-risk population not defined

    a.   Hospital records

         · Maternal deaths on maternity service
         · Maternal deaths on all services, including emergency room

    b.   Health worker surveillance or survey

    c.   Other: Church burials, newspaper reports, etc.

---

women and pregnancy outcomes, or (3) household surveys. The last two options
may be feasible only when maternal mortality rates are fairly high.

    Confidential enquiries into maternal deaths and their causes have been con-
ducted by physicians in the United Kingdom since 1949, and since the 1930s in some
states in the United States. This peer investigation process has probably been the
single most useful tool in understanding the cause of maternal deaths and in the
accurate classification of maternal deaths. However, when the investigation is
restricted to deaths from a passive surveillance system, such as vital statistics,
only the quality of causal information can be improved. The usefulness of confidential enquiries is augmented by including information from autopsies and demographic data from associated birth certificates for puerperal deaths. The latter
allows analysis of risk factor information, e.g. education and parity, which, in the
United States, is on birth but not on death certificates.

Active surveillance of maternal deaths is necessary to determine temporal relationships, to obtain complete reporting and to accurately classify maternal deaths so that we can identify priorities for intervention. In the United States national vital statistics detect only 83 percent of maternal deaths recognized by state health departments (Table 4). Moreover, state health departments, using death certificate surveillance only, detect only about 50 percent (Range 15–67 percent) of maternal deaths potentially identifiable through active surveillance. Detection of all maternal deaths requires active maternal mortality surveillance, including investigation of all deaths of women 12–49 or record linkage of pregnancy outcome events with deaths of women of reproductive age. In populations with high maternal mortality rates, other approaches, such as following cohorts of pregnant women (Khan, 1986; Alauddin, 1986) or household probability surveys, have been used successfully (Kwast, 1986).

Table 4: Comparison of Maternal Mortality Surveillance Procedures
in the United States and Selected Areas

| | Years | Deaths Detected | | Relative Completeness | Reference |
		(a)	(b)	a/b	
A. Vital statistics [National (a) vs. State (b)]	1974–78	1,949	2,349	83.0%	Smith, 1984
B. State vital statistics (a) vs. Maternal mortality committees (b)					
Massachusetts	1954–63	238	502	47.4%	Jewett, 1986
	1964–73	136	268	50.7%	
	1974–83	25	91	27.5%	
C. State vital statistics (a) vs. Hospital Surveillance (b)					
New Jersey	1974–75	30	52	57.7%	Ziskin, 1979
D. State vital statistics (a) vs. Record linkage (b)					
Georgia	1975–76	24	36	66.7%	Rubin, 1981
Washington	1977–81	17	36	47.2%	Benedetti, 1985
E. State vital statistics (a) vs. Investigating deaths of women 15–44 (b)					
Puerto Rico	1978–79	9	62	14.5%	Speckhard, 1985
Jamaica	1981–83	85	192	44.3%	Walker, 1986
F. Maternal mortality committees (a) vs. Investigating deaths of women 15–44 (b)					
Massachusetts	1981	8	10	80.0%	Sachs, 1984

WHO Maternal Mortality Tabulations

The World Health Organization's recently published tabulation of maternal mortality rates can be used to examine published maternal mortality for different parts of the world (see Table 5). The following comparisons do not take into account differences in definition and data collection. Reported annual national rates per 100,000 births for 1975−1984 range from two in Norway and Finland to 1,000 in three countries. For each of five regions at least one country--a high outlier--has a reported maternal mortality rate at least twice as high as the next highest rate. At least two of the eight outliers (Rumania, Paraguay) are known, through national statistics reported to WHO, to have had a major public health problem from abortion in 1973−76 (Table 6) (Tietze, 1983). Local studies suggest that Bangladesh and Mauritius also have high maternal mortality, at least in part, because of abortion-related deaths.

Maternal mortality rates in rural subnational areas in Africa and Asia (Table 7) suggest a median reported rate of 500−700 in both regions. These rates are substantially higher than the medians of national rates for Africa and Asia of 250 and 110, respectively. The rural rates may reflect more accurately the actual rates in these countries.

Table 5: Range of National Maternal Mortality Rates, by Region,
for Data Reported between 1975 and 1984

Region	Number of Countries	Range (excludes outliers)	High Outliers
Africa			
North	3	78−136	
West	7	84−530	
East	7	108−300	Somalia 1100
Middle	2	303−600	
South	1	200−300	
Americas			
North	2	6− 10	
Middle	7	65−103	
Caribbean	8	8−106	
Tropical South	9	65−216	Paraguay 469
Asia			
Southwest	5	5− 19	Democratic Yemen 100−1000
Middle South	6	80−150	Bangladesh 1500−3000
Southwest	7	5−300	
East	6	8− 50	Mongolia 100
Europe			
North	5	2− 4	Iceland 23
West	7	7− 25	
East	6	12− 22	Romania 175
South	6	10− 31	
Oceania	4	6− 47	Papua New Guinea 900
USSR	1	UNK	

Source: WHO, DFS, Maternal Mortality Rates 1985.
* Rate per 100,000 births.

Table 6: Fifteen Countries with Highest Reported
Abortion Mortality, 1973—1977

Country	Rate*
Romania	8.7
Paraguay	8.5
Mauritius	8.0
Chile	4.8
Trinidad & Tobago	4.6
Colombia	4.1
Guatemala	2.7
Ecuador	2.6
Venezuela	2.4
Barbados	2.0
Costa Rica	1.6
Uruguay	1.5
Philippines	1.3
Cuba	1.2
Nicaragua	1.1

Source: Tietze, C., Abortion Factbook, Table 20;
data from World Health Organization data bank.
* Per 100,000 women 15—44.

Table 7: Maternal Mortality Rates* in Rural Subnational Areas
in Africa and Asia, 1975—1983

Africa			Asia		
Area	Year(s)	Rate	Area	Year(s)	Rate
Gambia			Nepal		
Juli	1981-3	2,420	Dhankuta Dist.	1977	2,000
North Bank	1981-3	2,000			
			India		
Ghana			National	1978	1,360
National	1978	1,400			
			Bangladesh		
Tunisia	1975	1,000	Rural	1983	630
			Tangail	1982-3	570
Senegal			Matlab thana	1983	510
Sine Saloum	1983	700			
			Burma		
South Africa			National	1981	230
Umphambinyoni					
Valley	1983	550	China P.R.		
			Beijing	1982	30
Egypt					
Menoufia	1983	263 A+			
Tanzania					
So. Highlands	1983	153			

Source: Maternal Mortality Rates, WHO, Geneva, 1985.
* Rate per 100,000 births.

The value of 30 from a rural area in Beijing suggests China has achieved remarkably low maternal mortality; however, it is risky to extrapolate this rate from one local area to all of China. Moreover, in China, abortion-related deaths have not been included with maternal deaths.

I would like now to turn to three case studies. The first is Taiwan where adults, not health personnel, have registered births and deaths since the early 1900s.

Taiwan--A Case Study

Population-Based Investigation. One of the most comprehensive population-based investigations of registered maternal deaths in a lesser developed population was conducted in Taiwan in 1970 by the Institute of Maternal and Child Health (Fan, 1972). This investigation of maternal deaths based on household registration data was published in Chinese, not English, and is not well known. Before summarizing this study with some secondary analysis it is useful to know the extent to which maternal mortality had declined at the time of the study. The Taiwan Provincial Maternal and Child Health Institute (TPMCHI, 1981) reported a maternal mortality rate of 750 per 100,000 births in 1906, 651 in 1915, 490 in 1920, 380 in 1930, 310 in 1940, 197 in 1952, and 88 in 1962 (Figure 2). When it reached 62 in 1967 it was already less than 10 percent of the level which occurred 60 years earlier. It is worth noting that 50 percent of the decline occurred before 1930, or before the advent of hospitalized deliveries, blood transfusions, and antibiotics. This improvement has been attributed to the training of traditional birth attendants.

During 1971, two teams of public health nurses investigated 938 (81.1 percent) of 1,157 women who died while pregnant or during childbirth during 1965–1969. A typical woman who died was a poor illiterate housewife at least 30 years old who had had at least three children and had not used contraception. She had not received prenatal care because it was too far away. She delivered and died at home usually from rapid exsanguination following childbirth. One in 12 died from induced abortion.

Because the independent effects of age and birth order have been previously described in only two countries (England and Bangladesh), we present the age- and parity-specific mortality rates from this large data set in Table 8 and graphically in Figure 2. Overall the mortality rate was 6.4 deaths per 10,000 births. Mortality was lowest for women under 30 having their first, second, or third birth and highest for those age 30 or older who were having a fourth or higher order birth. Increasing age and parity appear to exert independent increased risk for maternal death. The cause of this increased risk has not been clarified by prior research.

In this study, adequate data on numerous risk factors were collected, but were not analyzed to show the relative risk of exposure to a condition--nor the association of risk factors with age and parity. One exception might be noted: for first births only one in seven women was illiterate, for eight and higher order births, four in seven were illiterate. For completed years of schooling, we can compute maternal mortality rates of 1.7 per 10,000 for college graduates, 2.0 for high school graduates, 3.9 for junior high school graduates, 6.0 for primary school graduates, and 7.6 for those with no schooling. Unfortunately the data do not allow one to determine the interaction between age, parity, and education.

Each of the following might be postulated to contribute to an increased risk among older, higher parity women: among all women who died, two-thirds did not have prenatal care, one-third had pre-eclampsia, one in 12 knew they had heart or kidney disease, one in five died from abortion (42 percent reported to be induced). For program planning, it would be useful to know the relative contribution of prior poor health or, inability to prevent unwanted pregnancy, lack of prenatal care, and lack of trained obstetric care to the extremely high mortality rate (2–3 percent) of

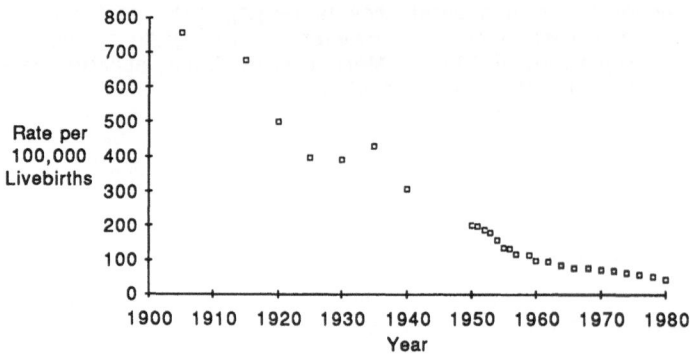

Fig. 2 Maternal Mortality Rates, Taiwan, 1906-1979.

Table 8: Maternal Mortality Rate* by Maternal Age and Birth Order,
Taiwan, 1965-1969

| Birth Order | Maternal Age | | | | | | | Total |
	15-19	20-24	25-29	30-34	35-39	40-44	45-49	
1	3.6	4.1	3.9	5.5	5.1	--	--	4.0
2	3.5	2.4	3.2	5.9	6.8	--	--	3.0
3	--	3.3	3.7	7.5	7.6	5.6	--	4.3
4	--	1.1	4.3	8.2	18.9	8.2	--	6.3
5	--	--	9.9	10.1	21.7	16.9	--	11.9
6	--	--	6.9	10.4	19.9	44.4	--	15.4
7	--	--	--	27.7	21.9	31.8	97.6	24.6
8	--	--	--	33.8	22.5	35.5	29.7	28.6
Overall	3.5	3.3	3.8	9.2	18.8	29.3	23.3	6.4

Adapted from Fan Guangyu, Ou Manmei, Investigative Report on the Causes of
Maternal deaths, Taiwan Institute of Maternal and Child Health: maternal deaths
adjusted for 18.9 percent of deaths lacking age or parity data; age and parity distribution of births based on registered births for 57 sample townships (19.6 percent
of all births) in Population Registration statistics in 1967.
* Rate per 10,000 births.

Unadjusted Number of Maternal Deaths

| Birth Order | Maternal Age | | | | | | | Total |
	15-19	20-24	25-29	30-34	35-39	40-44	45-49	
1	31	86	33	7	2	--	--	159
2	8	38	45	13	3	--	--	107
3	--	23	57	33	6	1	--	120
4	--	2	41	56	20	2	--	121
5	--	--	31	62	38	5	--	136
6	--	--	5	35	42	21	--	103
7	--	--	--	22	41	17	3	83
8	--	--	--	10	41	51	7	109
Total	39	149	212	238	193	97	10	938

older, high parity women. The correlation of illiteracy with high parity suggests the combination of social, economic, and biologic problems, and lack of health care among high risk women. Clearly, poverty was a major contributing risk factor.

By 1985, Taiwan had over 1,200 practicing obstetrician-gynecologists and over 90 percent of births occur under their attendance. Maternal mortality is now a rare event in Taiwan. It is however difficult to disentangle the contribution on maternal mortality of the direct effect of medical care and the indirect effect of social and economic improvement.

Lusaka, Zambia--A Case Study

Hospitals which provide virtually all maternity care for a defined population catchment area, such as a city, are uncommon but fortuitous sites for epidemiologic surveillance of maternal mortality. The University teaching hospital in Lusaka, Zambia, serves an estimated 85 percent of the maternity care to pregnant women in Lusaka. For 1982-83, 60 maternal deaths were investigated by hospital staff--a rate of 118 per 100,000 live births. (Mhango, 1986). This is the level of maternal mortality achieved by Blacks in the United States in the 1950s.

One-fourth of the deaths were due to abortive outcome, nine from an induced abortion. Hypertension, hemorrhage, and sepsis were the other three most common causes of death. The obstetrical staff judged 85 percent of the deaths to be avoidable. For the 58 percent which had a preventable performance factor associated with the hospital or staff, 71 percent occurred between 1600 and 0800 hours on the night medical shift. Fewer staff and more referrals of complicated cases during those hours contributed to the higher mortality at night time.

Improved child spacing and family planning services, better training for traditional midwives and continued maternal mortality surveillance by the obstetric staff to define and correct performance problems should lead to an accelerated decline in maternal mortality in Lusaka.

Bangladesh--A Case Study

The third case study is Bangladesh. The first population-based maternal mortality study was conducted in the late 1960s. Based on fewer than 50 maternal deaths, it showed an overall mortality of 500--600 maternal deaths/100,000 (Chen, 1975).

At least five population-based studies of maternal mortality have been conducted in Bangladesh since 1978. In 1978-79 Bangladesh Institute for Statistical Research and Training ascertained all maternal deaths known to 1,118 health workers in 63 hospitals and 732 non-hospital facilities (Rochat, 1981). Using data from Chen's study the authors estimated that health workers reported about 7.5 percent of the 21,600 women who died from pregnancy-related events that year. Moreover, only 3.6 percent were known to hospital personnel.

Eclampsia, induced abortion, hemorrhage, and obstructed labor were the four most commonly reported causes of death by both hospital and non-hospital personnel (Table 9). The widespread high level of mortality from induced abortion was unexpected.

A later prospective study of pregnant women in one rural community suggests that for every 40 women obtaining an abortion, one will die from complication of abortion. (Khan, 1986). These abortions are performed by traditional practitioners who most commonly place a stick or tree root into the cervix and leave it until abortion or death ensues. Induced abortion is a direct and, in this setting, often fatal consequence of unwanted pregnancy. The investigators concluded that at least one-fourth of maternal deaths could be prevented by "safe, effective, and acceptable means of fertility control, including contraception, menstrual regulation, and surgical sterilization."

211

Table 9: Frequency Distribution of Eleven Most frequent Causes of
Pregnancy-Related Deaths Reported by Hospital and Non-hospital
Personnel, Bangladesh, 1978—1979

	Hospitals	Non-hospital Facilities
Eclampsia	237	291
Induced abortion	201	297
Obstructed labor	87	137
Ante-partum bleeding	59	113
Post-partum bleeding	52	101
Retained placenta	30	111
Uterine rupture	35	51
Post-partum fever	20	45
Spontaneous abortion	6	28
Tetanus	16	3
Ectopic pregnancy	12	5
Other	60	93
Total deaths*	779	1,154

* Sum of columns exceeds totals because multiple causes of maternal
deaths, excluding abortion, were attributed to same death.

Three local area population-based prospective studies of pregnant women
conducted in 1983 showed no evidence for a decline in maternal mortality in Bangladesh (Khan, 1986; Alauddin, 1986; Koenig, 1986).

CONCLUSIONS

From these data we draw four concluding points:

1. World-wide maternal mortality is 99 percent preventable. The wide range of
death rates in each region of the world demonstrates that maternal mortality
can be markedly reduced in countries other than western industrialized
nations. All that is needed is strong national and international commitment to
maternal survival.

2. Unwanted pregnancies and induced abortion contribute heavily to preventable
causes of maternal mortality. Safe, accessible, and acceptable means of fertility control are an essential component of any realistic strategy to lower
maternal mortality.

3. The paucity of good population-based data on maternal mortality is appalling.
Since good data are often associated with good health care delivery, we infer
that a lack of data usually reflects high mortality and a lack of serious commitment to defining and reducing the problem.

4. Epidemiologic studies are needed to better determine the contribution of risk
factors (e.g., low education, lack of prenatal care, lack of safe water, sub-
stance abuse) for direct and indirect maternal deaths and the association, if
any, of pregnancy with nonmaternal causes of death, especially those due to
injuries, including homocide, suicide, and vehicular accidents.

ACKNOWLEDGMENT

The author thanks Dr. William Sappenfield for his contributions to this paper.

REFERENCES

Alauddin, M.   Maternal mortality in rural Bangladesh: The Tangail District. Studies in Family Planning 17(1):13, 1986.

American College of Obstetricians and Gynecologists (ACOG).   Standards for Obstetric and Gynecologic Services.   American College of Obstetricians and Gynecologists, Chicago, Illinois, 1974.

Atlanta Journal.   Teen is charged with deaths of 7 in house blaze.   The Atlanta Journal, 2-A, May 23, 1985.

Benedetti, T. J., Starzyk, P., Frost, F.   Maternal deaths in Washington State. Obstetrics and Gynecology 66(1):99, 1985.

Cates, W. C. Jr., Smith, J. C., Rochat, R. W., et al.   Assessment of surveillance and vital statistics data for monitoring abortion mortality, United States, 1972–1975. American Journal of Epidemiology 108:200, 1978.

Cefalo, R. C.   Memo: Final Report--Standard Terminology for Reproductive Health Statistics, June 12, 1985. American College of Obstetricians and Gynecologists, Washington, D.C., 1985.

Chen, L. C., Gesche, M. C., Ahmed, S., et al.   Maternal mortality in rural Bangladesh. Studies in Family Planning 5:334, 1975.

Fan Guangyu, Ou Manmei.   Investigative Report on the Causes of Maternal Deaths. Taiwan Institute of Maternal and Child Health (in Chinese), Taichung, Taiwan, 1972.

Jewett, J. F.   Maternal mortality. In B. P. Sachs, D. Acker, eds., Clinical Obstetrics: A Public Health Perspective. PSG Publishing Company, Littleton, Massachusetts, 1986.

Kaunitz, A. M., Hughes, J. M., Grimes, D. A., et al.   Causes of maternal mortality in the United States. Obstetrics and Gynecology 65(5), 1985.

Khan, A. R., Jahan, F. A., Begum, S. F.   Maternal mortality in rural Bangladesh: The Jamalpur District. Studies in Family Planning 17(1):7, 1986.

Khan, A. R., Rochat, R. W., Jahan, F. A., et al.   Induced abortion in a rural area of Bangladesh. Studies in Family Planning 17:95, 1986.

Koenig, M., Chowdhury, A. I., Faveau, V., et al.   Maternal mortality in Natlab, Bangladesh. Paper presented at 1986 Annual Meeting of the Population Association of America, San Francisco, 1986.

Kwast, B., Rochat, R., Widad, K. M.   Maternal mortality in Addis Ababa, Ethiopia: A household probability survey. Studies in Family Planning, in press, 1986.

Mhango, C., Rochat, R. W., Arkutu, A.   Reproductive mortality in Lusaka, Zambia, 1982-83:   An epidemiological analysis.   Studies in Family Planning, in press, 1986.

National Center for Health Statistics.   Annual summary of births, deaths, marriages, and divorces: United States, 1983. Monthly Vital Statistics Report 32(13):1, Hyattsville, MD: Public Health Service (OHHS Publication no. (PHS) 84-1120), 1984.

Rochat, R. W., Jabeen, S., Rosenberg, M. J., et al.   Maternal and abortion-related deaths in Bangladesh, 1978–1979.   International Journal of Gynaecology and Obstetrics 19:155, 1981.

Rubin, G. W., McCarthy, B., Shelton, J., et al.   The risk of childbearing reevaluated. American Journal of Public Health 71:712, 1981.

Sachs, B. P., Masterson, T., Jewett, J. F., et al.   Reproductive mortality in Massachusetts in 1981. New England Journal of Medicine 311(10):667, 1984.

Smith, J. C., Hughes, J. M., Pekow, P., et al.   An assessment of the incidence of maternal mortality in the United States.   American Journal of Public Health 74(8):780, 1984.

Speckhard, M. E., Comas-Urrutia, A. C., Rigau-Perez, J. Intensive surveillance of pregnancy-related deaths, Puerto Rico, 1978–1979.   Boletin Asociacion Medicine de Puerto Rico 77(12):508, 1985.

Taiwan Provincial Maternal and Child Health Institute. Statistics Relating to Maternal and Child Health in Taiwan (1979). Taichung, Taiwan, 1981.

Tietze, C. Induced Abortion: A World Review, Table 20. The Population Council, New York, 1983.

Walker, G. J. A., Ashley, D. E. C., McCaw, A. M., et al. Maternal mortality in Jamaica. The Lancet 486, 1986.

World Health Organization. Manual of the International Statistical Classification of Diseases, Injuries, and Causes of Death. World Health Organization, Geneva, 1977.

World Health Organization. Maternal Mortality Rates, a Tabulation of Available Information. World Health Organization, Division of Family Health, Geneva, 1985.

Ziskin, L. Z., Gregory, M., Kreitzer, M. Improved surveillance of maternal deaths. International Journal of Gynaecology and Obstetrics 16:281, 1979.

FUTURE POLICIES AND PRACTICES TO PROMOTE WOMEN'S HEALTH

Leila Mehra

Senior Medical Officer
Maternal and Child Health
World Health Organization
Geneva, Switzerland

First of all I should like to thank the organizers of the Christopher Tietze International Symposium for the privilege of delivering this closing keynote address. It seems quite appropriate that all of us who had a great regard for the late Dr. Christopher Tietze should be gathered here at this Symposium to honor his memory. Dr. Tietze will always be remembered for his internationally recognized work in the field of family planning, in promoting women's health and well-being through their right to and access to family planning. Further, we all recall his great friendliness and willingness to help those working towards this goal.

A very appropriate subject for me to present to you today is concerned with women's health especially with reference to reproduction, and about what we need to do in the future in order to improve the health of women in the world. I shall highlight some of the issues involved from a global point of view.

At the national level most countries (both developing and developed), and at the international level the United Nations and its specialized agencies like the World Health Organization (WHO), as well as non-governmental organizations and voluntary agencies are showing great concern, within the context of national and international cooperation, about the special health needs of women and about the key roles that women play in promoting health and development.

Countries have started to analyze the situation regarding women, health, and development; and action has been initiated at various levels, with an emphasis on the country level, to improve women's health and enhance their participation in health and development. The major obstacles and constraints to achieving full equity for women in the field of health and development are being considered and forward-looking strategies for the future activities proposed.

The year 1985 sees the close of the United Nations Decade for Women. For the past 10 years, the advocacy of women's roles and their needs has captured the public's attention all over the world and progress has been made. So why this focus on the future? Why are we not consolidating the general gains instead of redirecting our attention on women, health, and development?

One reason is that much of the progress has been patchy. Even the women in the industrialized countries, who led the drive for women's rights, have made gains that are at best limited. Regardless of whether women's lot is improving in one country or another, concrete strategies and plans to achieve greater gains are badly needed. Awareness of the need for further action is no more a by-product of the general women's movement; it is the result of a growing realization that women's health and their involvement in health care are essential keys to health for all. For women not only have their own special health problems relating to pregnancy and childbirth, but customarily they do most of the caring for their families. So if they are ignorant, malnourished, overworked, and have to bear large numbers of children beginning at an early age, the health of their families as well as their own health will suffer. This is especially true for the many millions of women who are confronted by illiteracy, poverty, poor sanitation, and medical and health care facilities that are inadequate or are physically or economically inaccessible.

While addressing the International Conference of Population in Mexico in August 1984, Dr. Halfdan Mahler, Director-General of the World Health Organization (WHO), said:

> When we talk of population, people appear as mere statistics. But it is people who matter; people who can make or break their own development. Some 1,000 million people are still trapped in poverty and underdevelopment. Is there any wonder that people in the developing countries should wish to act now? In 1977 WHO's Member States declared as the main social goal for the coming decades the attainment by the Year 2000 of a level of health permitting all to lead socially and economically productive lives. They decided that primary health care is the key to attain that goal, adopted a strategy, and are currently active in carrying it out. An essential feature of the strategy is the care of families, with particular emphasis on maternal and child health including family planning, and the status of women. Family planning can lead to striking improvements in the health of mothers and children and indeed the whole family.

> Attainment of health for all requires that governments, bilateral agencies, the United Nations system, and non-governmental organizations join forces in cooperative efforts in line with defined national policies which place health and well-being of people at the highest development ladder.

Almost a year later, in July 1985 in Nairobi, Dr. Mahler in his address at the World Conference to review and appraise the achievements of the United Nations Decade for Women, further emphasized:

> Health for all by the year 2000, adopted by the World Health Assembly, means a different approach by which health is considered in the broader context of its contribution to, and promotion by, social and economic development, so that all people including women will be able to lead socially and economically satisfying lives.

> What then, you might ask, has this to do with women's health and its development? In our health policies, isn't the health of mothers and children always at the top of our priority list? Doesn't the figure for maternal and infant mortality measure our progress in health development? Yes, I would reply-- but what about women?

> Women need to be considered for their own worth, as equal members of society, rather than as mothers, potential mothers or carers. They need to be seen beyond the limits of their contribution to family life, and they want to start sharing the responsibility for others, with the men in their lives and the men in the societies as a whole.

Clearly, if the goal of health for all is to be attained, more attention must be given to women's health and their roles in health and development. Forward-looking strategies are to be based on the recognition that women's health and their roles depend on broad considerations--including employment, education, and social status. Ultimately, they may even depend on equitable access to economic resources and political power. It is therefore imperative not to view the health aspects in isolation.

SITUATION ANALYSIS: WOMEN, HEALTH, AND DEVELOPMENT

Women's status is often described in terms of level of income, employment, education, health, and fertility, as well as their roles within the family, the community, and society. The biological and social realities of the maternal role are related to health status and are major factors in the problems women face in health, employment, education, and many other areas.

The value that society attaches to the maternal role is one of the crucial factors influencing the status of women. How do we react to an avoidable death during childbirth or to a child who is born too small to survive the first week because the mother's nutrition was so poor and her workload so great during pregnancy? Or to mothers who are unable to breast-feed because they cannot devote the time because of their jobs? Or to the lack of access to effective, safe and acceptable methods to regulate fertility? In short, how do we assess the social value accorded to reproduction and nutrition if women are denied the support needed to carry out these roles?

Reproductive Health and Family Planning

In most parts of the world women have a higher life expectancy than men. On average they live 7 years longer than men, but in many countries their biological advantage is cancelled out by discrimination in child care and lack of needed care during the reproductive years. Thus, in some parts of Asia and Africa, girls have a lower chance of survival up to the age of 5 years than boys.

An appalling number of women in the developing countries live in a chronic state of malnutrition, infection, and poor health linked to their low economic and social status. Little or no health care is available for conditions related to their reproductive health, especially pregnancy and childbirth. Complications of pregnancy and childbirth therefore account for a large proportion of deaths among women of reproductive age in the developing world. In certain developing countries, each time a woman becomes pregnant she runs a 200 times greater risk of dying than if she lived in a developed country. Failure to time and space pregnancies augments the risks of complications and death.

Most maternal deaths need not happen. Complications of pregnancy and childbirth--including hypertensive diseases (toxemia), obstructed labor, hemorrhage, and sepsis--are among the main causes of maternal mortality. Most of these deaths can be avoided by adequate maternal care.

Access to family planning services is the key to women's health and to their well-being in all aspects of their lives. Deprived of the means to plan their childbearing, women risk their lives in attempts to end undesired pregnancies. For example, in Latin America, half of all deaths among pregnant women are due to illegal abortion. Effective family planning can avoid such deaths.

Although most modern family planning methods have side-effects, real or perceived, the risks of these side-effects have to be weighed against the dangers of not using contraception, such as illegal abortions. In developing countries, a woman's chances of dying as a result of pregnancy are some hundred-fold higher than the chances of a woman using a modern contraceptive method dying from method-related causes.

217

In developed countries, a trained person is present at 98 percent of all birth, whereas in some developing countries, this is the case in 20 percent of births or less--even though it is crucial for all women to have proper care during their pregnancy and childbirth. Of the 128 million births taking place in the world each year, 58 million are still not attended by a trained person. One of the aims of primary health care is to ensure that every pregnant woman has access to skilled help.

While the majority of women in developing countries are deprived of life-saving health technologies for pregnancy and childbirth, in the developed countries women are now voicing serious concern about the abuse of technology and the over-medicalization of health care, in particular of pregnancy and childbirth, which imposes heavy human and financial costs on women!

Permanent Illness

Because they are not properly looked after in pregnancy and childbirth, millions of women are in a state of constant and debilitating ill-health which lasts for life. They can develop uterine prolapse, genital tract infections, fistula, and urinary incontinence. These conditions cause great physical and mental discomfort for the woman herself, and may lead the husband or the family to reject her, so that she becomes a social outcast.

Nearly two-thirds of pregnant women in developing countries--especially those who have pregnancies too close together--and half of all other women suffer from nutritional anemia. Malnutrition and anemia affect their psychological and physical health, lower their resistance to fatigue and disease and limit their working capacity, greatly increase the risk of illness and death in childbirth, and affect the health and birthweight of their offspring.

Women who do heavy work during late pregnancy gain less weight than others for the same food intake and they give birth to children of low birth weight, whose chances of survival or healthy growth are consequently reduced. Women often work a 12–16 hour day around the year, with seasonal peaks which add further stress. The resulting state of fatigue has major health effects on women and their children, especially in the case of women with sole responsibility for the family. The number of these women, left to cope alone with few resources or skills, is increasing rapidly among the urban poor in both developing and developed countries.

In many countries, girls complete only 2–3 years of schooling, although it is well known that educated women have healthier children. Education gives women a greater say in the family decision-making. Better education is also expected to be the means by which traditional practices harmful to women, such as nutritional taboos, female circumcision, and inadequate care for girls, will eventually be wiped out.

Cancer

Cancer of the cervix is the main female cancer in the developing world, where nearly 500,000 new cases occur every year (one in every 1,000 women aged 30–55 each year in Latin America). With early detection by cervical smear followed by treatment, the cure rate can be 100 percent; but these services are not yet widely available in the Third World. In developed countries the death rate from cancer of the cervix is the only death rate from cancer to have declined in the last 20 years.

Deaths from breast cancer--the most common female cancer worldwide-- have increased in industrialized countries reporting to WHO over the same period.

Also in industrialized countries, lung cancer deaths among women increased between 1960 and 1980 by a staggering 200 percent owing to the increased number of women who smoke. Changing lifestyles are also putting women at greater risk from alcohol dependence and cardiovascular diseases.

More and more women--like men--are working in industries where they are exposed to new chemicals and may ultimately suffer carcinogenic, mutagenic, or other toxic effects.

Health Care

Some 75 percent of all health workers are women, although they are rarely in a position to make decisions on health policy. Almost all traditional birth attendants and a large proportion of health care workers are women, and women predominate among hospital volunteers, at self-help clinics, and in other community organizations.

The proportion of female doctors is in the range of 3−30 percent in developing countries and 8−70 percent in developed countries. Very few female doctors hold positions of authority.

Women are also expected to look after the family's health, provide water and nutritious food, get children immunized, take them to the health services, and look after the sick and the elderly. Health care is therefore primarily a woman's field, but the quality of their participation has been limited by unequal access to training, information, education, and opportunities.

In traditional societies, women relied on each other and on the extended family for informal social support, but today--with changing family structures, more women working outside the home, and the loss of traditional means of support--much of the support women need to enable them to fulfill their many roles is not forthcoming.

Governments can help improve women's and children's lives by legislative measures, such as maternity leave and breast-feeding breaks, and by adopting policies of social support to women. Increasingly, governments are recognizing the potential of nongovernmental organizations and women's informal networks, and are turning to them both for advice, and active contribution to health and health-related programs.

Maternal Mortality and Family Planning

Women are the main victims of unregulated fertility. Maternal mortality rates--the risk of dying from pregnancy-related causes--vary greatly in different parts of the world. In Europe today, the rates are as low as 6 per 100,000 live births compared with rates up to 1,000 per 100,000 live births reported in parts of Africa and Asia. Moreover, not only do women in the world's poorest countries undergo the highest risk of dying from a given pregnancy--due to their own poor health and to the lack of appropriate care--but they also undergo this risk more frequently and over a longer period of their lives than women in developed countries. Without family planning they will continue childbearing for 20 or even 25 years, while women in industrialized countries typically have two or possibly three children spaced over 5 or 10 years. Unregulated fertility, high rates of illegal abortions, and partial or total absence of care during pregnancy and childbirth are main reasons for the fact that every year over half a million women in developing countries die during pregnancy and childbirth, leaving at least one million children motherless. Most of these maternal deaths are preventable and family planning has a crucial role to play in this prevention.

Illegal abortions kill up to 200,000 women a year and permanently injure the health of countless more. When couples have access to effective methods of contraception, women do not need to resort to dangerous illegal abortions in order to control their fertility. The high number of abortions thus provide a clear indication of the unmet needs and desire to practice family planning.

Birth Spacing Reduces Child Death Rates
and Improves Child Health

Recent findings in several developing countries confirm that children born after intervals of less than 2 years have a significantly higher mortality than children born after longer intervals. Children born less than one year after the end of their mother's last pregnancy are more than twice as likely to die than children born after an interval of 2 years or more. Estimates for developing countries show that if all births were at least 2 years apart, infant mortality could be reduced by an average of 10 percent and 1-4 years child mortality by around 16 percent. A significant proportion of infants born in developing countries are disadvantaged from birth through low birth weight, caused by the poor health and nutritional status of the mother whose condition has been aggravated by repeated childbirth. Infants born after a short interval since the mother's previous pregnancy are particularly prone to low birth weight. It is estimated that out of approximately 125 million annual births in the world, roughly 20 million are low birth weight (i.e., one in six births), with a higher risk of death and a lower potential for health, growth, and development.

Family Size and the Outlook for the
Health of Mother and Child

The number of children a woman conceives affects her chances of having safe and successful pregnancies and deliveries. From the sixth child on, prospects become less favorable with each additional pregnancy. Birth order is clearly related to infant and young child mortality. Children of birth order seven or more have mortality rates one-third higher than those of birth order two or three. Children of high birth orders are likely to be born to mothers who are older and physically exhausted. They will have to compete with older brothers and sisters for food, attention, and love, and are often cared for by someone other than the mother, often an older sister. Children from large families often have more frequent illnesses and grow more slowly than those from smaller families.

Early and Late Childbearing
Have Their Dangers

Infant and maternal mortality are highest among teenage mothers. Women who become pregnant while they are still adolescent have a much higher risk of complications during pregnancy and childbirth. These complications can injure their health or even cost them their lives. Fetal deaths are least common among children born to women between the ages of 20 and 35. Children born to women who are teenaged are at increased risk of premature birth and those born to women older than 35 run a much greater risk of birth defects and a higher risk of infant and maternal mortality. In some countries a considerable portion of first births occur to young women under 20. Postponing the first birth--whether by marrying at a later age or by suitable family planning--will greatly improve a woman's health status, make pregnancy and childbirth less hazardous, and give the baby a healthier start in life and the mother a chance to mature physically, mentally, and emotionally.

Breast-Feeding Helps to Regulate Fertility

In addition to its physiological and psychological advantages for the newborn baby, breast-feeding delays the return of fertility and thus lengthens the interval before the next pregnancy. In rural and traditional societies in the developing world, breast-feeding, especially 'on demand' feeding, actually plays a major role in spacing births. If it were to decrease greatly or disappear, the contraceptive services needed to compensate for that loss would be considerable. For example, if in one developing country with almost universal breast-feeding the pattern of breast-feeding were to change to that typical of industrialized countries a few years ago to maintain fertility at current levels, a more than five-fold increase in contraceptive use, from 9 percent to about 52 percent, would be required. Regarding individual families wanting to space or limit their pregnancies, traditional methods such as breast-feeding have however to be complemented by the use of technically and culturally appropriate contraceptive methods.

Family Planning Also Serves the Infertile Couple

In some parts of the world infertility affects a large number of couples, causing deep unhappiness. Family planning, as part of maternal and child health, has a role to play in enabling such couples to become parents. The purpose of family planning is not merely contraception, but to help the couple to have the number of children they want, when they want them. This means also helping the infertile couples.

Family Planning and the Status of Women

The status of women, in particular their level of education, is closely related to fertility and mortality patterns. Quite apart from the possible health effects of family planning, the ability of couples to regulate their own fertility has opened the way for women to achieve the full and equitable participation in social and economic development that is their due.

The Unmet Need for Family Planning Services

About 95 percent of the people in the developing world live in countries which provide some form of public support to family planning programs, generally as part of maternal and child health programs. Despite this, it has been estimated that there are about 300 million couples who do not want any more children but who are not using any method of family planning, chiefly due to inadequate access to services in the developing world, especially in rural areas and urban slums.

As always, the poorest layers of the population are the last ones to be provided with social services. The primary health care movement provides a unique opportunity to extend essential health care, including maternal and child health and family planning, to all families and communities and thus it enables millions of couples who would like to plan their families to avail themselves of the necessary advice and care. To be effectively used, modern methods of contraception not only need to be relevant to sociocultural beliefs, customs, and patterns but also have to be backed up by the health and medical services and by supervision, which primary health care services can provide together with trust and confidence in health workers.

The Unmet Need for Improved Methods of Fertility Regulation

If women the world over were able to have the children they say they want, the crude birth rate would range between 16 and 28 per 1,000 population rather than the present range of between 28 and 40. In many countries, couples use no method of contraception at all or resort to traditional methods and illegal abortion. Many modern contraceptive methods have some side-effects, both real and perceived, but the health risks of unwanted and unplanned pregnancies to the mother and the child might be far greater than the risk of the side-effects of these contraceptives. Nevertheless, many couples and some health workers are reluctant to use or recommend existing contraceptive methods. Accordingly, there are unmet needs for new and improved contraceptive methods, including improved oral contraceptives, long-acting agents, vaginal rings, new barrier methods, modern male methods, as well as improved methods for natural family planning.

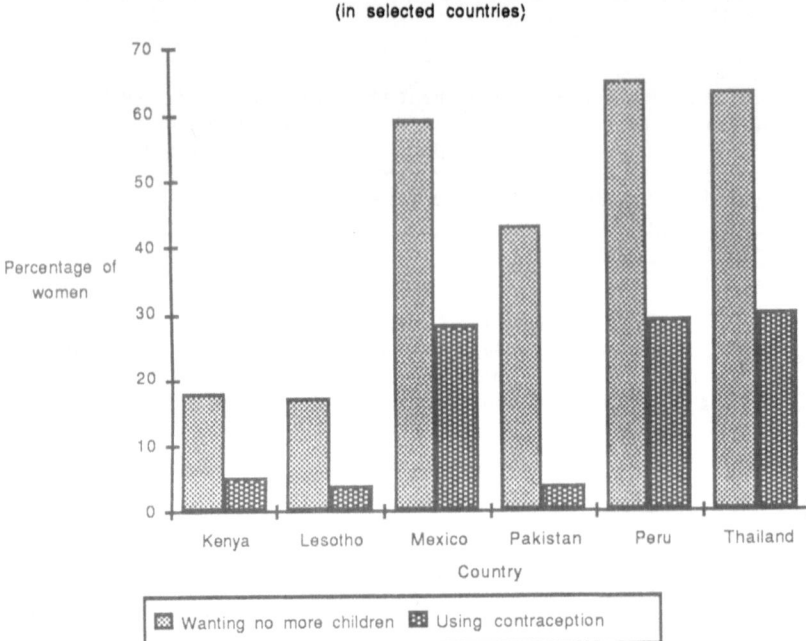

Fig. 1. Women and Family Planning.

Information Support and Transfer

Accurate and adequate information, relevant to local circumstances, is essential for appropriate action. Country averages for specific indicators often mask inequalities between population groups such as geographical areas as well as between sexes. Thus it is important to have, as far as possible, data disaggregated according to population groups.

Despite the special importance of local data, countrywide information can be useful for assessing the general scope and nature of problems. Some countries have done a great deal of research concerning women (particularly in the last 5 years), and others are just beginning their efforts in this direction.

Information on particular topics related to women's health is also increasing, governments are reporting studies on the prevalence of anemia and other nutritional deficiency diseases, low weight gain in pregnancy, and the distribution of food within the family and its effect on the nutritional status of women and girls.

At the global level, information has been gathered on a variety of specific topics such as female mortality and the prevalence of nutritional anemia. At the global level, WHO has established a clearing house to collect and provide information and material for WHO programs and women's organizations throughout the world.

Publications have been prepared which (a) highlight specific women's issues within a program area; (b) describe women's health issues as a whole, combining existing information from all program areas; and (c) describe certain health problems from a woman's perspective.

Throughout this mechanism a large number of key persons and institutions regularly receive these and other information. This also includes preparation and distribution of an information kit on women, health, and development in collaboration with the Joint United Nations Information Committee.

Primary Health Care for Women's Special Needs

The principles of primary health care and total coverage provide a framework for reaching women in greatest need. Of particular relevance is maternal and child care, including family planning. Evidence indicates that, although the situation may be improving, there is still a long way to go. Countries are increasingly recognizing the need for more active measures to make such care available. A review of international financial and technical resources currently being applied to the improvement of the health of women and children in developing countries indicated that 30 percent of funds allotted to health are devoted to various aspects of maternal and child health, including family planning.

Over-utilization of technology and over-medicalization of pregnancy and childbirth have become a major problem in developed as well as in urban areas of developing countries. For example, fetal monitoring in some countries has resulted in an increase in the number of caesarian births owing to errors in readings. Sociocultural relevance as well as women's perceptions are important considerations for the appropriate and successful use of technologies.

Social Support Measures for Women

Recent studies on breast-feeding highlight the importance of women's living conditions for children's nutrition and health, and recent research on women's roles indicates the complexity of the situation everywhere for poor women who have to work in order to ensure family survival.

In traditional societies women have relied on each other and their extended families for informal social support. However, considerable unmet needs are arising where family structures are changing, increasing numbers of families are depending on women's incomes for survival, and women are losing their traditional means of support.

Governments can give support by means of policy decisions and legislative action that provide adequate maternity leave and facilities for breast-feeding among working mothers.

Other important legislative measures are those governing the minimum legal age of marriage; women's rights in marriage and in cases of divorce, rape, and abortion; harmful traditional practices; basic constitutional guarantees of equality, including equal pay for equal work. Occupational health risks for women, particularly regarding reproductive health, are receiving attention. The crucial role that governments can play in providing social support to women is undeniable. But even in some developed countries the underlying assumption is that difficulties arising from the combination of motherhood and employment (formal and informal) are to be borne solely by the individual. Women, having been excluded from most formal organizations and networks, have developed their own informal systems and approaches to problem solving. In almost all countries there are women's networks which form a natural community-based mechanism for action. Governments are increasingly recognizing the contribution these groups and organizations make, as well as their potential, and are seeking their aid and advice.

Women's organizations have special characteristics that make them a key factor in community involvement and an ideal entry point and partner in primary health care facilities. They are traditionally supportive, motivated, and interested in health care; able to understand and carry out intersectoral activities basic to primary health care; have a positive attitude towards voluntary work; and are acceptable both to the family and the community.

The grass-roots organizations' main goal is usually to satisfy the immediate needs of their members as they see them, the purpose of intermediary organizations is to support local groups like self-help groups as well as their own membership. They often work from urban centers, and may be motivated by religion, profession, politics, or business.

International women's organizations and associations or federations of national nongovernmental organizations reflect the social or political biases of their national affiliates. Because of their international standing and prestige they provide important links between the community organizations and the government.

Women as Health Care Providers

In an effort to better understand and improve the status of women as health professionals a number of country-based projects are being undertaken essentially as an action-oriented and problem-solving effort.

Intersectoral Activities

Many governments have established offices, commissions, or ministries to serve as a coordinating mechanism for women's affairs in intersectoral programs.

An interagency Task Force on Women and International Drinking-Water Supply and Sanitation Decade (IDWSSD) is collaborating in efforts to improve community water supply and sanitation through recognition of the role of women and promotion of women's participation in IDWSSD activities at national, regional, and international levels.

FORWARD-LOOKING STRATEGIES: POLICIES AND PRACTICES

The national, regional, and global forward-looking strategies for the advancement of women's health and women in development are an elaboration of health-for-all strategies. The goals for health-for-all through the primary health care approach are so closely aligned with the interests of women that their achievement would by definition meet the particular health needs of women and enable them to contribute fully to the health of the family, community, and nation.

Before turning to opportunities and strategies for the future, let us examine a few of the obstacles and constraints (as discussed in some detail earlier in the text) that must be overcome if full equity in health and development has to be achieved.

A major constraint to progress has in fact been a lack of awareness of the extent and seriousness of the problems.

The enactment of legislation and policies is perhaps the second greatest area of change during the decade. Major gaps, however, remain between the spirit of the law and its implementation.

The amount of resources devoted to the implementation and enforcement of policy changes bears little relation to the political commitment expressed.

There is a lack of mechanisms for increasing the participation of women in health endeavors at all levels and for drawing women into decision-making, thus bringing them into the mainstream.

There is also the male's reluctance to share family responsibilities.

Let us now look at an outline of the forward-looking strategies which indicate the measures necessary to overcome obstacles and constraints and build upon the important activities already under way.

1. National Strategies

Each country must analyze the situation of women at the local and national levels to determine the relevant major issues. Each community, country, and regional grouping of countries must select its own priorities, and try to achieve what is feasible in a socioculturally relevant manner within the context of its particular possibilities, resources, and constraints. The strategies highlight approaches that would make a substantial contribution to progress not only for women, but for all people, and indicate a way of thinking concerning the integration of women's issues within health programs.

The regional strategies are based on priorities identified within the regions that would support country needs and actions. The global strategies, in turn, are designed to provide maximum and appropriate support to the regions and countries in their efforts to improve the situation.

2. Health Science and Technology

The following strategies are proposed with regard to the essential elements of primary health care:

a. Education concerning prevailing health problems and methods of preventing and controlling them:

- ensure that messages meant to be received by women are relevant to their health priorities and are suitably presented

- ensure that education is geared towards changing social attitudes and values that are discriminatory against women and detrimental to their health (e.g., attitudes against child spacing)

- ensure that women have access to appropriate health education

b. Promotion of an adequate food supply and proper nutrition:

- facilitate women's access to adequate nutrition for themselves and their children

- foster activities that will increase awareness of the special nutritional needs of women, especially during pregnancy and while breast-feeding

- promote the provision of social support during pregnancy and while breast-feeding

c. Adequate supply of safe water and basic sanitation:

- ensure that women are consulted with regard to technologies used in water and sanitation projects (e.g., in selecting pumps that are not too heavy for them to operate and durable enough to withstand continual use)

- provide support to local women's groups to include water and sanitation activities in integrated programs

d. Maternal and child health care, including family planning:

- provide technical and methodological support to strengthen the maternal and child health and family planning component of primary health care; increase emphasis on the assessment, adaptation, development, and field-testing of acceptable family planning methods and appropriate technologies addressing problems specific to pregnancy and delivery

- support traditional practices that enhance the health of women and children (e.g., breast-feeding) and discourage harmful practices

- promote fertility patterns that are not detrimental to women's health and that of their children, and the provision of appropriate information and services for family planning, including infertility

- provide family planning advice and services, appropriate to the cultural setting, to adolescent girls to avoid precocious childbearing, which is harmful to women's health

- promote behavioral and nutritional patterns that foster healthy pregnancies

- prevent and treat complications of pregnancy and childbirth

- promote social support measures that will facilitate women's economic and family roles, such as day care for children, maternity leave, and breast-feeding breaks, as well as care of the elderly

- follow up recent recommendations of the World Population Plan, which reaffirmed the need to take measures to control mortality and morbidity, and to this end enhance the status of women in health and development through maternal and child health and family planning

- give special attention to technologies for priority areas of women's health, in particular with a view to overcoming abuses and overuse of technologies in pregnancy and childbirth and ill effects of contraceptives

- promote intersectoral activities that especially affect the health of women and children

e. Immunization against the major communicable diseases:

- collect and analyze information on immunization, according to sex

- ensure that pregnant women are, or have been, immunized against tetanus

f. Prevention and control of locally endemic diseases:

- ensure women's full participation in prevention and control programs for communicable and noncommunicable diseases (e.g., in the family and through women's groups and organizations)

- develop and/or adapt socially relevant technologies, where necessary, for prevention and control

g. Appropriate treatment of common diseases and injuries:

- ensure that services are conveniently located

- ensure that services are available at times and on days of the week that are suitable for women, bearing in mind their work patterns

- ensure that services can be afforded by women

- ensure that the training of health workers includes education on the true nature and value of women's contribution to health care

h. Provision of essential drugs:

- ensure that essential drugs are relevant to women's health needs and priorities

- ensure that essential drugs specific to the health needs of women are available in the health facilities

- prevent misuse of drugs that could be harmful to women's health or to the health of their offspring

i. Prevention of mental disorders and promotion of mental health in women:

- give special attention to the psychological factors that are important for women in relation to the utilization of health services (e.g., attitude of health workers, health care settings)

- devise ways of assessing the needs of special groups of vulnerable women (e.g., migrants, women whose husbands have migrated, and the urban poor), and promote measures for dealing with those needs (e.g., self-help and other community groups)

- promote research on the relationship between the mental health and psychosocial problems of women and development

3. Health System Infrastructures

Information gathered for evaluating health situations and trends and health systems should be suitable for assessing women's health needs. Data on morbidity and mortality should therefore be collected and analyzed according to sex, and sex-specific socioeconomic indicators should be included in monitoring progress towards health for all.

Managerial processes for national health development should take women's issues into account, and women should be involved in all stages. Strategies are to:

- establish mechanisms for collaboration between various health services, health institutions, and nongovernmental and voluntary organizations, with special emphasis on women's organizations

- ensure that women are equitably represented at decision-making levels

Health systems research should be integrated within the managerial process, taking women's issues into account. Strategies are to promote research on:

- problems faced by women regarding the utilization of health services

- women's roles as health care providers in the home and community

- the relationships between health and women's work and time patterns

- the integration of health activities within women's development programs

- the influence on health of social, economic, and behavioral factors specific to women

- the development of appropriate technology and evaluation of their effectiveness, safety, and acceptability

Health legislation facilitating the attainment of health objectives specific to women should be promoted. Strategies are to promote legislation to:

- protect maternity (e.g., paid maternity leave)

- prevent the abuse of women's bodies (violence, sexual exploitation, sexual mutilation)

- ensure working conditions for women which promote good infant and young child health and nutrition

- prevent occupational hazards specific to women

- prevent abuses of technologies regarding women's health

- control the marketing of substances harmful to women's health

- provide back-up community support measures for women

- fix a minimum age for marriage that is safe for childbearing

Appropriate health care facilities should be planned, constructed, and equipped so as to be readily accessible and acceptable to women—in harmony with their work and time patterns as well as their needs and perspectives.

Women are key human resources in the formal health care system. Strategies to redress existing imbalances and to raise the status of women as health professionals are to:

- ensure that women and men have equal training for all levels of health care and are equally remunerated

- redress imbalances in the proportions of women in certain health professions

- promote the training of women for managerial positions

Among the principles and approaches of primary health care and health-for-all that are particularly relevant to women, two stand out as being especially important: community involvement and intersectoral approaches.

4. Community Involvement

Communities in general, and women in particular, are already very actively involved in making decisions about their own health care and disease prevention.

Education should be provided to women and women's organizations to make them aware of their rights and responsibilities for their own personal health care and that of their families, and to encourage them to demand health services that will meet their particular needs and concerns. Strategies to support women's organizations in health care activities are to:

- devise ways of involving women and women's organizations in decisions concerning the health system, at all levels

- ensure that women's organizations are represented in national and local health councils or committees

- encourage women's organizations to promote and participate in activities

- encourage local women's organizations to participate in primary health care in their communities

- devise ways of supporting women in taking responsibility for self-care as well as community care

- take steps to change men's attitudes so that health care responsibilities, especially in the family, are shared by women and men

- encourage young girls to be involved in health activities

5. Intersectoral Approaches

These are to:

- enact social policies that ensure equity in all aspects of development

- enact policies that will give women the social and economic freedom to space their children and limit the size of their families

- establish mechanisms for intersectoral action, such as the representation of government departments responsible for women's affairs in multisectoral health councils and interministerial committees

- provide resources, including small amounts of "seed money," to women and women's organizations at the grass-roots level to enable them to organize intersectoral activities

- support intermediary-level community groups in carrying out activities such as: fundraising for local projects; training and education programs; providing facilities for local groups' actions, etc.

6. Global Strategies

At the global level, the following strategies are proposed:

- provide technical support for incorporating a women's dimension in ongoing programs at all levels

- develop women's components of intersectoral programs related to health

- promote the involvement of women's organizations in primary health care

- support country reviews of existing roles of women's organizations in health, including maternal and child health/family planning

- support and liaise with women's nongovernmental organizations at international, regional, and national levels

- collect and collate information on women's health issues

- increase knowledge and understanding about how the various socioeconomic factors related to women's status affect and are affected by their health

- increase resources for women's health

- facilitate women's health care roles

- promote equality in health development

7. Monitoring Progress

Significantly, many of the global indicators for monitoring progress towards health-for-all are of direct relevance to women and can be used to monitor progress in women's health and their participation in health development at the global and national levels--e.g., the proportion of infants with a birth weight less than 2,500 g (indicator of nutrition and health in pregnancy); access to trained personnel

229

Table 1: Global Health-for-All and Other Indicators Relating to Women, Health, and Development (by United Nations geographical region; about 1982)

Region	WHO Global Indicators				Others			
	(1) % Adults Literate Male/Female	(2) % Births Attended by Trained Personnel	(3) % Infants Low Birth Weight	(4) Infant Mortality Rate Male/Female	% Enrolled in School		(7) % Women Aged 15–19 Married	(8) Average Number of Children per Woman
					(5) Aged 6–11 Male/Female	(6) Aged 12–17 Male/Female		
WORLD	67/54	56	16	103/92	76/64	55/46	30	3.8
Developed	98/97	98	7	24/18	94/94	84/85	8	2.0
Developing	52/32	49	18	116/104	70/53	42/28	39	4.4
AFRICA	33/15	33	14	151/129	59/43	39/24	44	6.4
Northern	44/18	30	10	128/114	70/45	42/43	34	6.2
Western	20/6	39	17	171/145	44/30	29/16	70	6.8
Eastern	29/14	26	13	142/121	55/41	33/20	32	6.6
Middle	35/9	24	16	181/153	78/54	52/26	49	6.0
Southern	55/56	66	12	109/92	82/86	74/70	2	5.2
NORTH AMERICA	99/99	100	7	16/12	99/99	95/95	11	1.8
LATIN AMERICA	76/70	65	10	90/80	78/78	58/54	16	4.5
Middle	75/67	49	12	76/67	84/83	58/46	21	5.3
Caribbean	67/66	60	12	78/68	85/87	60/59	19	3.8
Tropical South	74/67	70	9	104/92	70/72	56/54	15	4.6
Temperate South	93/91	88	7	47/41	98/98	70/73	10	2.9
ASIA	56/34	51	20	108/99	73/54	43/28	42	3.9
Southwest	58/31	51	7	123/99	78/57	54/32	25	5.8
Middle South	44/17	24	31	138/135	70/44	35/17	54	5.5
Southeast	75/53	52	17	105/87	71/65	43/35	24	4.7
East	97/92	94	6	57/45	99/99	85/80	2	2.3
EUROPE	96/93	97	7	25/19	95/96	81/80	7	2.0
Northern	99/99	100	6	15/11	98/98	82/83	9	1.8
Western	98/98	100	5	17/13	95/96	87/89	5	1.6
Eastern	97/92	99	8	30/21	92/91	80/81	9	2.3
Southern	93/85	93	7	31/25	97/97	73/66	7	2.3
USSR	100/100		8	35/27	99/99	72/82	10	2.4
OCEANIA	90/88		12	48/39	88/87	75/71	10	2.8

Sources: Columns 1, 5, and 6—UNESCO; columns 2 and 3—WHO estimates; columns 4, 7, and 8—Population Reference Bureau and United Nations Population Division.

for attending pregnancy and childbirth; and female literacy (a potent indicator of women's status, with a strong influence on their own health and that of their families, their fertility, and their participation in health development).

Several other global indicators, if collected separately for each sex, would provide useful indications concerning women's and girls' health status—e.g., infant mortality, immunization coverage, weight-for-age, and life expectancy.

There are many other powerful indicators that can be used at the country level: of these, none is more telling than maternal mortality. Fertility rates, birth intervals, the proportion of first births taking place to very young women (under 18 years) or to older women (over 35 years), and availability or use of contraceptives are all good indicators of women's control over their own lives. Nutritional status indicators include data on weight-for-height, the prevalence of nutritional deficiency diseases, especially anemia, and weight gain in pregnancy. Minimum legal age at marriage and/or the proportion of teenage women married, and the proportion of girls enrolled or attending school, are all status indicators directly related to health (Table 1). The involvement of women and women's organizations at the primary health care level is important, but statistics on the proportion of women at the policy and decision-making level in the health sector are a better indicator of women's equitable participation.

As to infant mortality, it should be noted that biological and prenatal conditions of the mother particularly affect the mortality in the first months of infancy, and continue to affect morbidity and health status of both boys and girls in later life.

The above-mentioned indicators that are already included in the monitoring of progress towards health-for-all will provide a basis for assessing the situation of women and improvements over time. In addition, however, countries use other indicators appropriate to their specific needs. Some of these, mentioned above, would better reflect the special health needs of women, as well as their roles in health and development in a given situation; as an integral part of a country's monitoring, they would add significantly to the baseline of information of particular relevance to the health status of women and, in view of women's key role in health, of the whole population.

The close of the United Nations Decade for Women must therefore be viewed only as a beginning. Much more remains to be done!

REFERENCES

Mahler, Dr. H., Director-General of WHO. Address at the World Conference on Population, Mexico City, August 1984.
Mahler, Dr. H., Director General of WHO. Women and health for all. Address at the World Conference to Review and Appraise the Achievements of the United Nations Decade for Women, Nairobi, July 16, 1985.
WHO. Women, Health, and Development: A Report by the Director-General, World Health Organization. Offset Publication No. 90, Geneva, 1985.
WHO Media Service. Health and Family Planning. In Point of Fact No. 23, 1984.
WHO Media Service. Women and Health. In Point of Fact No. 27, July 1985.

Latin America (continued)
  illegal abortion
    cost of, in, 67·
    incidence of, in, 12
    mortality in, 13, 20, 217
  population growth in, 71, 199
  sterilization in, 8
Legislation, see Abortion law
Lewit, Sarah, 27, 120
Life expectancy for women, 217
Lung cancer, 218

Malaria, 203
Malaysia, 9
Malnutrition, 217
Malta, 18
Maternal and child health, 61, 120, 216,
    223
Maternal mortality, see Mortality,
    maternal
Mauritius, 207
Medroxyprogesterone acetate (Depo-
    provera), 199
Menstrual regulation (MR)
  in Bangladesh, 111
    availability of, 116, 155, 157
    complications of, 116, 154, 155
    costs of, 160, 161
    definition of, 111, 154
    incidence of, 111, 112, 154, 155
    reporting of, 112
  in Malaysia, 163
  training in, 76, 111, 114, 115, 117,
    154
Menstruation, 49
  implants and, 40
  irregular, 33, 40, 48
Mexico, 70
Middle East, 12
Morbidity, see Abortion, complications
  of
Mortality, infant, 68, 70, 73, 74, 89, 94,
    95, 111, 120, 216, 220, 230,
    234
Mortality, maternal, 69, 60, 71, 74, 77,
    86, 93, 111, 201, 207—209
  abortion and, 12, 13, 14, 20, 59, 65,
    70, 74, 86, 89, 178
  in Africa, 13, 207, 219
  in Asia, 207, 219
  in Bangladesh, 111, 151, 153, 207, 211
  causes of, 204, 209—211, 212, 217,
    219
  childbirth related, 13, 14, 89
  in China, 208
  decline in, 13, 89, 93—95, 120, 209
  definitions of, 202, 203
  in developing countries, 199, 204, 217
  in Europe, 219
  gestation and, 12, 13

Mortality, maternal (continued)
  illegal abortion and, 13, 57, 59, 69,
    92, 151, 153, 169, 199
  in India, 74
  in Korea, 65
  in Latin America, 70, 71, 86, 199
  in Nigeria, 57
  in Paraguay, 207
  in the Philippines, 169
  risks of, with contraceptive methods,
    27, 29
  in Rumania, 207
  sources of data on, 204, 212
  surveillance of, 206, 209, 211
  in Taiwan, 209—211
  in the United States, 120, 178, 201,
    206
  worldwide, 13, 201, 207, 212
  in Zambia, 211
Myomata, 143, 165, 166

National Abortion Federation (NAF),
    119, 120, 142, 191, 193
Netherlands, 8, 18, 20, 47, 83, 86, 87,
    183, 185
New York State, 12, 106, 175
New Zealand, 11, 18—20
Nigeria, 14, 53—60
  abortion law in, 53—55
  attitudes toward abortion in, 55, 56
  attitudes toward fertility and
    marriage in, 57
  contraceptive use in, 58
  illegal abortion
    incidence of, in, 55
    reasons for seeking, in, 56, 57
    resulting in sepsis, in, 56, 57
  maternal mortality in, 57
  sexual activity in, 55, 56, 58
Non-governmental organizations (NGO),
    155, 161, 188, 215, 216
Norgestrel, 32
Norplant^R, 39—42, 199 (see also
    Hormonal implants)
Norway, 18, 20, 207

Obstructed labor, 211, 217
Oral contraception (pill)
  antibiotics and, 49
  criticisms of, 5, 24, 49
  failure rate of, 11, 46—48
  labelling of, 29
  post-abortion use of, 165, 198
  post-coital use of, 31, 32, 35
  progestin-only (minipill), 24, 39, 48
  use effectiveness of, 5, 24, 48
Osmotic dilators, see Cervix, dilation
    of; Dilators)
Oxygenation, 144

Panama, 67, 70